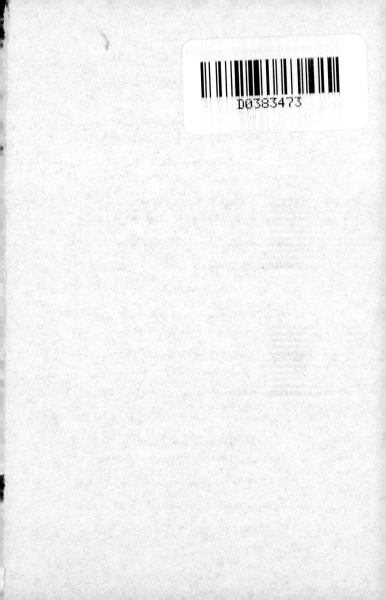

OUR
MALADY

OUR
MALADY

Lessons in Liberty from a Hospital Diary

TIMOTHY SNYDER

CROWN
NEW YORK

A Crown Trade Paperback Original

Published in the United States by Crown, an imprint of
Random House, a division of Penguin
Random House LLC, New York.

CROWN and the Crown colophon are registered trademarks of
Penguin Random House LLC.

Library of Congress Cataloging-in-Publication Data
Names: Snyder, Timothy, author.
Title: Our malady / Timothy Snyder.
Description: New York: Crown, [2020]
Identifiers: LCCN 2020024457 (print) | LCCN 2020024458
(ebook) | ISBN 9780593238899 (paperback; alk. paper) |
ISBN 9780593238905 (ebook)
Subjects: LCSH: Medical care—United States.
Classification: LCC RA412.3 .S64 2020 (print) |
LCC RA412.3 (ebook) | DDC 362.10973—dc23
LC record available at https://lccn.loc.gov/2020024457
LC ebook record available at https://lccn.loc.gov/2020024458

Printed in the United States of America on acid-free paper

crownpublishing.com

2 4 6 8 9 7 5 3 1

Book design by Caroline Cunningham

First Edition

For now we see through a glass, darkly;

but then face to face: now I know in part;

but then shall I know even as also I am known.

FIRST CORINTHIANS 13:12

CONTENTS

Prologue: Solitude and Solidarity   3

Introduction: Our Malady   13

Lesson 1. Health care is a human right.   19

Lesson 2. Renewal begins with children.   61

Lesson 3. The truth will set us free.   81

Lesson 4. Doctors should be in charge.   111

Conclusion: Our Recovery   135

Epilogue: Rage and Empathy   143

Acknowledgments   147

Notes   149

OUR
MALADY

Solitude and Solidarity

When I was admitted to the emergency room at midnight, I used the word *malaise* to describe my condition to the doctor. My head ached, my hands and feet tingled, I was coughing, and I could barely move. Every so often I was seized by tremors. The day that had just begun, December 29th, 2019, could have been my last. I had an abscess the size of a baseball in my liver, and the infection had spilled into my blood. I did not know this at the time, but I knew that something was deeply wrong. *Malaise*, of course, means weakness and weariness, a sense that nothing works and nothing can be done.

Malaise is what we feel when we have a malady. *Malaise* and *malady* are good old words, from French and Latin, used in English for hundreds of years; in American Revolutionary times they meant both illness and tyranny. After the Boston Massacre, a letter from prominent Bostonians called for an end to "the national and colonial malady." The Founding Fathers wrote of malaise and malady when discussing their own health and that of the republic they founded.

This book is about a malady—not my own, though mine helped me to see it, but our common American one: "our public malady," to borrow James Madison's phrase. Our malady is physical illness and the political evil that surrounds it. We are ill in a way that costs us freedom, and unfree in a way that costs us health. Our politics are too much about the curse of pain and too little about the blessings of liberty.

When I got sick at the end of last year, freedom was on my mind. As a historian, I had spent twenty years writing about the atrocities of the twentieth century, such as ethnic cleansing, the Nazi Holocaust, and Soviet terror. Recently I have been thinking and speaking about how history defends against tyranny in the present and safeguards freedom for the future. The last time I was able to stand before an audience, I was giving a lecture about how America could become a free country. I hurt that evening, but I did my job, and then I went to the hospital. What followed has helped me to think more deeply about freedom, and about America.

When I stood before the lectern in Munich on December 3rd, 2019, I had appendicitis. That condition was overlooked by German doctors. My appendix burst, and my liver became infected. This was neglected by American doctors. That is how I ended up in an emergency room in New Haven, Connecticut, on December 29th, bacteria racing through my bloodstream, still thinking about freedom. In five hospitals over three months, between December 2019 and March 2020, I took notes and made sketches. It was easy to grasp that freedom and health were connected when my will could not move my body, or when my body was attached to bags and tubes.

* ❦ ❦

When I look at the pages of my hospital journals, stained by saline, alcohol, and blood, I see that the New Haven sections, from the last days of the year, concern the powerful emotions that rescued me when I was near death. An intense rage and a gentle empathy sustained me, and provoked me to think anew about liberty. The first words I wrote in New Haven were "only rage lonely rage." I have felt nothing cleaner and more intense than rage amidst deathly illness. It came to me in the hospital at night, giving me a torch that ignited amidst kinds of darkness I hadn't before known.

On December 29th, after seventeen hours in the emergency room, I had an operation on my liver. Lying on my back in a hospital bed in the early morning hours of December 30th, tubes in my arms and chest, I couldn't ball my fists, but I imagined that I was balling my fists. I couldn't raise my body from my bed on my forearms, but I had a vision of myself doing so. I was one more patient in one more hospital ward, one more set of failing organs, one more vessel of infected blood. But I didn't feel that way. I felt like an immobilized, infuriated me.

The rage was beautifully pure, undefiled by an object. I was not angry at God; this was not His fault. I was not angry at the doctors and the nurses, imperfect people in an imperfect world. I was not angry at the pedestrians moving freely about the city beyond my chamber of twisted sheets and tubes, nor at the deliverymen slamming their doors, nor at the truckers blowing their horns. I was not angry at the bacteria celebrating the bounty of my blood. My rage was directed against nothing. I raged against a world where I was not.

I raged therefore I was. The rage cast a light that revealed an outline of me. "The shadow of the solitary is the unique," I wrote, rather obscurely, in my diary. My neurons were just starting to fire. The next day, December 31st, my mind began to recover from the sepsis and the sedation. I could think for more than a few seconds at a time. My first extended thought was about uniqueness. No one had ever moved through life as I had, making just the same choices. No one was spending New Year's Eve in exactly the same predicament with just the same emotions.

I wanted my rage to lead me out of my bed, and into another year. In my mind's eye I saw my dead body, its decomposition. The predictability of rot was horrible. It is the same for everyone who has ever lived. What I wanted was unpredictability, my own unpredictability, and my own contact with the unpredictability of others.

For a few nights, my rage was my life. It was here, it was now, and I wanted more of the here and more of the now. In my bed I craved a few more weeks, and a few more weeks after that, when I wouldn't know what would happen to my body, wouldn't know what would play out in my mind—but would know that the person feeling and thinking was me. Death would extinguish my sense of how things could and should be, of the possible and beautiful. It was against *that nothing*, "that particular nothing," as I wrote in my diary, that I raged.

The rage was with me for only a few minutes at a time, bringing warmth as well as light. My body usually felt cold, despite my fever. In my hospital bed on New Year's Eve I wanted the sun to come up, and I wanted it in the room. I wanted it on my skin. After three days of trembling, I needed more than my own warmth, which escaped through the thin sheets that kept twisting around the tubes in my chest and arm. The winter sunrise in New England through a thick window isn't much; I was living in symbols and desires.

I didn't want the torch in my mind to be a lonely light. And it was not. People came to visit me. My wife opened the shade, and the wan New Year entered. When other visitors began to arrive, I guessed how they would react at bedside to a helpless me, but I didn't know. I remembered that some of the old friends visiting me think that patients who are visited get better treatment. They are surely right: health is a matter of being together, in that way and a hundred others.

A visit helps us to be alone. Being together in solidarity permits a return to solitude in tranquility. Just by appearing, my friends set off memories, chains of association back into our past. I remembered a moment when one friend had shared that pragmatic view of why patients should be visited: years before, when it was I who was at her bedside, when it was she who was ill, and pregnant, in the same hospital where I myself now lay. I thought about her children, then about mine. Another mood was coalescing: a gentle empathy.

❋

The rage was pure me, my wish to be a sound not an echo, to compose not decompose. It was not against anything, except the entire universe and its laws of unlife. For a night or two I could shine in my own light.

Yet, slowly and softly, a second mood impinged, one that sustained me in a different way: a feeling that life was only truly life insofar as it was not only about me. Like the rage, this mood visited me when I was alone, when I could do little for myself, when my whole sense of motion came from visions in my mind. In this mood I felt myself to be in a cluster of something with other people, tumbling through time. When I tried to draw the feeling in my journal, I came up with an uneven, floating conveyance. It looked a bit like a raft.

A raft can be built over time from bits and pieces. I was a part of a raft, and others were, too; we were floating and jostling together in the same water, sometimes effortlessly, sometimes against the rocks. If my plank fell into the deep, the raft might lose its way or capsize. Some planks of the raft were further from mine, and some were closer. I recited to myself the ways my children's lives were bound to my own. What mattered was not that I was distinct, but that I was *theirs: their father*. Every bit of their existence involved the expectation of my presence. They had never not touched me. Their planks had always been bound to mine.

I imagined what would change without me, beginning with the daily details that mark the mental calendar of a parent: soccer practice, math homework, reading out loud. I recognized with pain that my vision of my son without me, of my daughter without me, were just as real as my previous life with them. I watched their future unfold without me, in my mind's eye, and then I reeled it back.

This floating recognition that my life was not my own, this gentle empathy, escorted me away from death. This sense that life was shared began with my children but extended outwards, an uneven collection of timber making up the raft. I was splashing and tugging forward with everyone I knew and loved, and all would be affected if I fell away now. In this mood I was not raging, but floating along, remembering, contemplating, empathizing.

The rage helped me see myself, helped my body and mind take on distinct form after a shock. The empathy placed me among others. In this mood, it was not so important that I was special. It was important that I was inside other people, in their memories and expectations, a support in the shape of their lives, a buoy during difficult passages. Since my life was not just my own, then my death was not just my own. When I reached that point, I began to rage again. This could not happen.

The empathy, though altogether different from the rage, worked together with it. Each mood revealed a truth, an element of me. Neither was enough; I needed both. I needed the torch and the raft, the fire and the water, the solitude and the solidarity, to get well, to be free. And what is true for me, I suspect, is true for others.

INTRODUCTION

Our Malady

Had I died, my death would have been all too typical, a passing into sad statistics. Far too many Americans needlessly departed life in the early months of 2020. Far too many Americans are too close to death every month, every moment. Although we have been promised ever longer lives, life expectancy in our country has flatlined, with no meaningful change in half a decade. In some recent years the life expectancy of Americans has declined.

The beginning of life in this country is frightening and uncertain. Care of expectant mothers is wildly uneven and grossly inadequate. Black women often die in childbirth, and so do their babies. The mortality rate of babies borne by African American women is higher than in Albania, Kazakhstan, China, and about seventy other countries. America as a whole does worse than Belarus, the most Soviet of the post-Soviet states; and Bosnia, an awkward creation of the Yugoslav civil wars—not to mention forty other countries. Young adulthood has lost its charm. Unless something changes, millennials will live shorter lives while spending more money on health care than Gen-X parents or boomer grandparents. The prime of life is not what it once was. Middle-aged white men are committing suicide and drugging themselves to death in astonishing numbers. Middle-aged white women in the South are dying before their time.

Our system of commercial medicine, dominated by private insurance, regional groups of private hospitals, and other powerful interests, looks more and more like a numbers racket. We would like to think we have health care that incidentally involves some wealth transfer; what we actually have is wealth transfer that incidentally involves some health care. If birth is not safe, and is less safe for some than for others, then something is wrong. If more money is extracted from young adults for health care, but they are less well than older generations, something is wrong. If the people who used to believe in the country are killing themselves, something is wrong. The purpose of medicine is not to squeeze maximum profits from sick bodies during short lives, but to enable health and freedom during long ones.

Our malady is particular to America. We die younger than people in twenty-three European countries; we die younger than people in Asia (Japan, South Korea, Hong Kong, Singapore, Israel, Lebanon); we die younger than people in our own hemisphere (Barbados, Costa Rica, Chile); we die younger than people in other countries with histories of British settlement (Canada, Australia, New Zealand). Other places keep passing us in the longevity charts. In 1980, when I was ten, Americans lived on average about a year less than inhabitants of countries of comparable wealth. By 2020, when I was fifty, the difference in life expectancy had grown to four years. It is not that other countries have more knowledge or better doctors. It is that they have better systems.

The gap between the United States and other countries grew in 2020, since no democracy mishandled the coronavirus pandemic as we have done. People in

Japan and Germany, in South Korea and Austria, and indeed in all rich democracies, were at less risk than we were, because their governments treated them better, and because they had better access to information and care. It was already far too easy to die in this country before the novel coronavirus arrived in the United States. Our botching of a pandemic is the latest symptom of our malady, of a politics that deals out pain and death rather than security and health, profit for a few rather than prosperity for the many.

The new coronavirus ought to have been taken seriously from the time of my hospitalization, which is when it was documented. In January 2020 we should have acquired a test for the novel coronavirus, tracked the new disease down, and limited its reach. This could easily have been done. Far poorer countries did it. Americans infected with the coronavirus should all have had access to hospital beds and ventilators, and the doctors and nurses who treated them should have had enough masks and gowns. A virus is not human, but it is a measure of humanity. We have not measured up well. A hundred and fifty thousand Americans are dead for no reason at all.

Our malady makes pollution deaths, opioid deaths,

prison deaths, suicides, newborn deaths, and now mass graves for the elderly all too familiar. Our malady goes deeper than any statistic, deeper even than a pandemic. There are reasons why we are living shorter, unhappier lives. There are reasons why a president thought he could keep Americans ignorant during a pandemic, and exploit our confusion and pain. Our malady leaves us isolated, uncertain where to turn when we hurt.

America is supposed to be about freedom, but illness and fear render us less free. To be free is to become ourselves, to move through the world following our values and desires. Each of us has a right to pursue happiness and to leave a trace. Freedom is impossible when we are too ill to conceive of happiness and too weak to pursue it. It is unattainable when we lack the knowledge we need to make meaningful choices, especially about health.

The word *freedom* is hypocritical when spoken by the people who create the conditions that leave us sick and powerless. If our federal government and our commercial medicine make us unhealthy, they are making us unfree.

Freedom is sometimes a scream in the dark, a will to go on, a solitary rage. I needed that in my hospital bed. But a person wanting to be free over the course of a life also needs calm voices, friendly visits, confidence that illness will bring attention and not abandonment. That, too, helped me make it alive into a new year, our year of pandemic. The lessons I sketch here, arising from thoughts and experiences I jotted down in my hospital notebooks, are about how solitude and solidarity work together.

Freedom is about each of us, and yet none of us is free without help. Individual rights require common effort. The Declaration of Independence posits that "all men are created equal," and closes with the willingness of all of its signatories to defend that principle. A right is something that we are convinced we deserve, but it only becomes real in the world when forced upon the powers that be.

"The whole history of the progress of human liberty," as Frederick Douglass reminds us, "shows that all concessions yet made to her august claims have been born of earnest struggle." It will be a struggle to heal our malady. The struggle begins when we claim health care as a human right.

LESSON 1.

Health care is a human right.

I was in Germany when I got sick. Late at night in Munich on December 3rd, I was admitted to a hospital with abdominal pain, and then released the next morning. In Connecticut on December 15th, I was admitted to the hospital for an appendectomy and released after less than twenty-four hours. In Florida on vacation on December 23rd, I was admitted to the hospital for tingling and numbness in my hands and feet, but released the following day. Then I began to feel worse, with a headache and growing fatigue.

On December 27th, we decided to return to New Haven. I had not been satisfied with treatment in Florida, and I wanted to be home. But it was my wife, Marci, who had to make the decisions and do the work. On the morning of the twenty-eighth, she packed everything up and got our two kids ready to go. I was a burden. I had to lie down to rest after brushing my teeth and after putting on each article of clothing. Marci arranged for wheelchairs at the airports and got us where we needed to be.

At the Fort Myers airport I sat in a wheelchair with the children on a curb while she returned the rental car. As she remembers the journey, "You were fading from life on the flight." At the Hartford airport she wheeled me from the plane straight to a friend's car, and then stayed with the kids to wait for the luggage. Our friend had not known what was happening; she took a look at me in the wheelchair, said "What have they done?" in Polish, and got me into the front seat. I lay down flat as she sped to New Haven, because my head hurt less that way.

I struggled to get admitted to the emergency room in New Haven. I had to use a wheelchair to get from the parking lot to the lobby of the emergency department. Another friend, a doctor, was waiting for me there. Although I did not understand this then, I had a massive infection in my liver, which was leaking into my bloodstream. I was in a condition known as sepsis; death was close. The nurses guarding the entrance to the emergency room did not seem to take me seriously, perhaps because I did not complain, perhaps because the friend who advocated for me, though a physician, was a black woman. She had called ahead to say that I needed immediate treatment. That had no effect.

After the better part of an hour sprawled between a wheelchair and a table in the lobby, I finally got into the emergency department. Nothing much happened then, so I reflected on what I had seen as I stumbled from the lobby to an emergency room bed. I have been in many emergency rooms in six countries, so I have a feel for them. Like most American emergency departments, this one was overflowing, with beds lining the hallways. In Florida six days before, the overcrowding had been even more severe. I felt lucky in New Haven that night to get a small area to myself: not a room, but a sort of alcove separated by a yellow curtain from the dozens of other beds outside.

After a while, the curtain started to bother me. Getting attention in emergency rooms is a matter of figuring out who staff are and catching someone's eye. I couldn't see people passing when the curtain was closed, and so it was hard to decipher the uniform colors and the name badges and ask for help. The first doctor who opened the curtain decided that I was tired, or perhaps had the flu, and gave me fluids. My disconcerted friend tried to suggest that my condition was something more serious. "This is someone who was running races," she said. "And now he cannot stand up." My friend told the resident that this was my second emergency room visit within a few days, so extra attention was warranted. The resident left unconvinced, and with the curtain partway open behind her. I caught a glimpse then of the two nurses who had admitted me, and heard what they said as they passed: "Who was she?" "She said she was a doctor." They were talking about my friend. They laughed. I couldn't write this down then, but did later: racism hurt my life chances that night; it hurts others' life chances every moment of their lives.

In New Haven, as in the rest of the country, emergency departments in the evening are full of older alcoholics and younger people who have been stabbed or shot. Saturday nights in New Haven are tough, for doctors, nurses, staff, and patients. This was a Saturday night. Trying to stop my violent trembling, I pulled the sheets up, and recalled another Saturday night in this same emergency department, a scene that had played out in the next alcove over.

About eight years before, I had come to the emergency room with my pregnant wife after she had cut two fingers badly while slicing bread. She was two weeks from her due date, and less than usually coordinated. I heard the scream, rushed downstairs, tried to staunch the bleeding, and called 911. The ambulance crew was visibly worried about domestic violence. They found us on our knees on the floor of the kitchen, blood everywhere, me holding Marci's hand above her heart and explaining quietly to our two-year-old son what was happening. Seeing this posture, the paramedics moved very slowly and asked questions in practiced, controlled voices.

In the ambulance with my wife, the paramedics loosened up and said our boy was cute. I waited at home with my son until some friends could come and take him for the night, then joined my wife in the emergency department. We waited several hours for a specialist, apparently because some of the plastic surgeons did not want to brave the emergency room on a

Saturday night. Ours was relieved that the fingers were not severed, which is what he had been expecting in the time and place. As we left the building, we realized that my wife had left a scarf wrapped around the corner of her bedframe. I trotted back to get it, only to find a pair of handcuffs on the rail where the scarf had been, attached to the wrist of a man with a more serious knife wound. He had the scarf around his neck. I let it be.

In the early morning hours of December 29th, expiring slowly in the emergency room alcove, I had plenty of time to remember. I was tested, slowly, for flu, for this and that, with little result. I had undergone my appendectomy in the same hospital two weeks earlier, but no one in the emergency department seemed inclined to look at my electronic record. I had brought a folder with the printouts and a CD from the Florida hospital, and I had just enough presence of mind to offer it to the doctors. They were not interested. "We do things our own way," said the resident. The doctors and nurses seemed unable to complete a sentence, let alone think about my case as something with a history.

I could see, or rather hear, why they were distracted. The familiar sounds from beyond the curtain drew my attention as well, even as my vital signs worsened and the infection spread through my blood. An alcoholic beyond the curtain to the right, an older lady from the sound of her voice, kept crying out "Doctor!" or "Nurse!" A second alcoholic, to the left, was a loquacious homeless man. When asked for his belt, he riffed on the idea of the "Belt of Orion," comparing himself to the hunter and rapist of Greek mythology. Whenever approached by a female doctor or nurse, he said, "You belong to me; don't try to fight it." One of the nurses declared that she didn't belong to anyone. When he was discharged, he was asked the standard questions about whether he felt safe at home. This was absurd, since he had no home and was going back out into the cold. It was also obscene, since his answers to the questions involved the sexual violence he imagined perpetrating upon the nurse who was asking them.

Two policemen sat just beyond the curtain, observing two wounded young men. With nothing much to do, the cops moved closer together, just in front of my curtain, and loudly talked the night away. I learned how the police department organizes its shifts. I heard stories of drunk driving, abandoned vehicles, domestic assault, and, the favorite theme, rumbles in the open air that the police were powerless to stop. Some of the stories were funny, like the one about the woman who was caught, shovel in hand and dirt on her knees, undoing the gardening work of her neighbor.

The two police officers preferred different topics: the one bureaucracy, the other criminality. The one who liked to talk about crimes used the terms *unperson* and *unpeople*. In George Orwell's novel *1984*, an *unperson* is someone whose memory has been expunged by the state. It seemed, though, that the policeman had in mind African Americans he regarded as criminals. I wanted to speak to him about that, but lacked the strength.

I was fading. After three hours in my alcove my fever reached 104. My blood pressure crashed: 90/50, 80/40, 75/30, 70/30. I was hanging somewhere in between. Sepsis kills people, and mine was not being treated.

While I was in this suspended state, the sounds from beyond the curtain never ceased. My senses took it all in, my brain formed the words uttered by everyone around me, but I was no longer mediating the stimuli. I was not in charge, or there was not enough left of me to be in charge. The policemen's conversation kept coming through, as did the drunken shouts, the squeak of shoes on the floor, the wheeze of an automatic door, the slap of a hand on the button that opened it, the knock of a bed against it. The curtain to my alcove followed the bodies of people passing by, or danced with a draft from beyond.

❦

When I closed my eyes in the early morning hours, I could still see the moving curtain. The rippling became hypnotically regular, from right to left, like an invertebrate sea creature undulating with the waves. The color of the curtain deepened from yellow to ochre. An inky black around the edges replaced the fluorescent white of the lights outside.

For five hours, from about one to about six in the morning on December 29th, I had trouble remaining conscious. Each time I closed my eyes the rippling ochre curtain beckoned. I tried to keep them open. The blood pressure reading behind me provided a point of focus. Each time I turned back from my vital signs towards the curtain, though, I would eventually have to close my eyes. Then the color of the curtain would change to ochre, its movements would become darkly voluptuous, and I would remember.

My whole life did not rush before my eyes. It was rather that my ability to suppress memories dissolved. A few images of childhood came on heavy, with punching force. I could no longer induce them to make way for other memories or for new thoughts. It was strange to be a spectator of the real, rather than a referee.

The memories of adulthood were less about what befell me and more about what I learned from others. When I concentrate on what I read, I have a very good memory. Much of my thirties and forties I spent reading first-person accounts of the Holocaust and other German crimes, Stalinist mass shootings and famine, ethnic cleansings, and other atrocities. These came now, too, unbidden, a thousand jabs: one after the other, book after book, document after document, photograph after photograph.

A Ukrainian boy asks to starve to death in the open air rather than in underground barracks. A Polish officer hides his wedding ring so that it will not be plundered when he is murdered. A Jewish girl leaves a message for her mother scratched on the wall of a synagogue: "We kiss you over and over." Something in me paused over a Jewish orphan taken in by childless Ukrainian peasants: "You will be like a daughter to us," they said, she remembered, I remembered. Something in me hesitated over the story of a woman whose special gift, as she hid Jews in her apartment, was to behave as if nothing extraordinary were taking place. Poise. Existential poise. A certain photograph I had looked at regularly for twenty-five years appeared before my eyes again: a Polish Jew named Wanda, full of self-possession. Wanda had refused the German command to go to the Warsaw ghetto in 1940 and kept her two boys safe throughout the war. Her husband, their father, was murdered.

It went on, the black and white of remembered words and images, the ochre curtain rippling in the background, neither near nor far, neither on this side nor that. I was with others. At first I was uneasy with the society of the dead, but this passed. I had learned from them. In some way I remembered what they remembered. Wanda's younger son grew up to become a historian, who approved my dissertation fifty-five years after his mother had saved him from the ghetto.

Twenty years after that, I found the record of what his mother had done, and wrote about it myself. Life is not just inside people; it passes through people.

It was the ochre curtain I didn't like; it was the passage into death, repulsive and attractive, that I feared. I never drew it in my diary; I remember it all too well.

❦ ❦

My body was not well cared for during the early hours of December 29th. Fluids brought my blood pressure up some, but no meaningful treatment took place. The doctors and nurses could not spend more than a few seconds at a time with me, and rarely made eye contact. They ran their blood work, forgot the results, misreported them, ran off. The permanent distraction of doctors and nurses is a symptom of our malady. Each patient has a story, but no one is following the story.

Two weeks earlier, at the time of my appendectomy, other doctors had noted a lesion in my liver, but had neglected to treat it, or examine it again, or order another test, or even mention it. I had been discharged from the hospital the day after that surgery, December 16th, with too few antibiotics and no information about that second infection. When I was admitted to the hospital in Florida on December 23rd with tingling and numbness in my limbs, I had not known to tell the doctors about my liver. Again I was discharged after a day. In the emergency room in New Haven on December 29th, everyone dismissed the possibility that my condition had to do with my appendix or my recent surgery. It seemed unthinkable to the doctors in New Haven that their colleagues had done something wrong. This sort of clan thinking is an elementary error, the kind we all make under stress.

The doctors in New Haven did think that the doctors in Florida might have made a mistake. As it became clear that I had some kind of bacterial infection, they suspected meningitis arising from a spinal tap performed in Florida. The New Haven doctors therefore performed a second spinal tap, but were distracted even as they punctured my back and searched for the spinal fluid. The resident made an obvious mistake, penetrating my spine through the wound of the previous puncture, which is to say at the putative site of infection. The attending physician had to tell her to pull the needle back out. People are much poorer at almost every task when they are close to a cell phone;

both physicians had kept theirs turned on and close by. I was hunched over a bed with my face against a wall; I know this because their cell phones rang three times during the procedure. The first was the most memorable. After reinserting the long needle in my spine at a second point, the resident jumped in reaction to her ringtone. Bent over the railing of my bed, I did my best not to move.

My body was at the mercy of the permanent distraction of doctors. My friend had called the surgeon who performed my appendectomy; she did not remember the liver finding and did not, at this or any other time, mention that it was in the record. If the attending physician and the resident in the emergency department hadn't been distracted, they could have taken a moment to look at the record of my previous surgery themselves, noted the liver problem, and spared me the second spinal tap. If they had been able to talk to me for a moment longer, I could have shown them my Florida record, which indicated elevated liver enzymes, an important clue to what was happening. I had even circled those results on the paper, but I couldn't get anyone to pay attention to them. If the two doctors had silenced their cell phones before the spinal tap, they could have done what they thought they needed to without shaking the needle in my spine. Like everything that happened, this wasn't my bad luck. It is the nature of the system that doctors are harried and make mistakes.

I was in sepsis for a long time. Britain's National Health Service recommends that antibiotics be administered to a septic patient no later than one hour after admission. My father-in-law, a physician, was trained that the doctor should see to this personally. In my case I had to wait eight hours, until after that surreal second spinal tap. Nine hours after that test's negative result, the curtain was drawn, and my bed was pulled from the alcove into an operating room. Someone had finally looked at my scans from the time of the appendectomy and noticed the neglected liver problem. A new scan then showed that the abscess in my liver had grown very large during the two weeks it was ignored. After an urgent procedure to drain my liver, I was wheeled to a hospital room, the one where I would spend the last two days of 2019 and the early part of 2020—where I raged and empathized. After my post-operative care was mishandled, I underwent another procedure on my liver, to add two more drains.

33

I was released weeks later with nine new holes in me: three from the appendectomy, three for liver drains, two from spinal taps, and one in my arm for the tube that channeled the antibiotics I was to inject. My hands and feet were still tingling, my neurologist now believes from nerve damage caused by my immune system when it reacted to an overwhelming threat.

As I write, I am still in treatment: taking medication, undergoing tests, and seeing doctors. For me, writing is part of the treatment, because my own malaise has meaning only insofar as it helps me understand our broader malady. I remember places where I should not have been, things that should not have happened, not to me nor to anyone else, and I want to make sense of them.

After I was discharged from the hospital in New Haven, I heard that colleagues were astounded that my wife and I hadn't called in powerful patrons to protect me when I was in the emergency room. That had not occurred to us. If the system does work that way, it should not. If some Americans have access to health care thanks to wealth or connections, they will feel pleased because they are included and others are not. Such a feeling turns our human concern about health into a silent yet profound inequality that undermines democracy. When everyone has access to decent care at minimal cost, as is true for almost all of the developed world, it is easier to see fellow citizens as equal.

Part of our malady is that there is nothing in our country, not even life and not even death, where we take the proposition that "all men are created equal" seriously. If health care were available to everyone, we would be not only healthier physically but also healthier mentally. Our lives would be less anxious and lonely because we would not be thinking that our survival depended on our relative economic and social position. We would be profoundly more free.

Since health is so elemental to existence, confidence about care is an important part of freedom. If everyone can assume that treatment will be available when necessary, they can turn their minds and their resources to other matters, make freer choices, pursue greater happiness. If, on the other hand, people think that care is preferential, then those who are on the inside start to take pleasure from the suffering of those who are on the outside. If health care is a privilege rather than a right, it demoralizes those who get it and kills those who do not. Everyone is drawn into a sadistic system that comes to seem natural. Rather than pursuing happiness as individuals, we together create a collective of pain.

And so our malady concerns us all. We all take part in the collective of pain. Those of us who are doing better are harming those who are less well-off. When health care is competitive the winners do wrong to others, but they also get worse care themselves. Distracted by their relative advantage, they do not see that by harming others they are also harming themselves. If health care were a right, we would *all* have better access to treatment, and would all be liberated from the collective of pain. Health care should be a right, not a privilege, for the sake of our bodies, and for the sake of our souls.

🍂 🍂

In the days between my release from the hospital and the closure of the buildings of my university due to the coronavirus pandemic, I went to my office. I wanted to make a copy of my hospital diary and put it in a safe place.

I looked around at the chaos of years of work and travel, the piles on the tables, the books on the floor: it all seemed a bit strange to me after the months away. I felt compelled to put everything in order. I was too weak to do much else: a few books shelved, a few files sorted, and I had to lie down. As I stepped back from death, I was looking for easy ways to bridge the gap between what I wanted to do and what I could do, and getting my library and my documents in order was one. In moving paper around I also wanted to put memories back in their places. I wanted the ochre curtain out of my mind. I wanted control of what I saw when I closed my eyes.

When I rested and looked at my shelves, I began to reconsider the experiences of people I had written about, the victims and survivors of mass murder. I have written books about policies that directly, and without ambiguity about intentions, took human life: shooting, starving, gassing. It occurred to me—as it has occurred to others long before me—that the deliberate deprivation of health was a related harm. People could be treated as inhuman sources of disease rather than as fellow humans to be treated and cured. People could be sorted by health and worked to death in the name of some greater good for some other group.

One shelf in my office is devoted to Nazi Germany

and the Holocaust. A book there collects the correspondence, writings, and speeches of Adolf Hitler. In Hitler's first antisemitic letter he referred to Jews as "racial tuberculosis." In the middle of an influenza epidemic, Hitler was calling human beings a contagion. After Hitler came to power, Nazis accused Jews of spreading disease among a healthy German population. During the Second World War, Nazis called Jews "typhus bacteria." Confining Jews in ghettos without medical care did in fact make them sick. German tourists who visited the ghettos made a spectacle of malady. As Jews fell ill, Nazis treated that as an argument for killing them quickly. Hitler boasted of cleansing Europe of Jewish bacteria, of "lancing the boil."

If we think that the Nazi Holocaust is the depth of malevolence, what then is the height of good? If we decry Hitler's language and actions, what follows for what we ourselves say and do? The Nazis treated health care as a way to divide the humans from the subhumans and nonhumans. If we see others as bearers of ailments and ourselves as healthy victims, we are little better than they. If we truly oppose the Nazi evil, we will try to think our way to its opposite, to the good. A part of that effort is to understand that all humans are subject to malady, and have an equal claim to care.

Another shelf of books in my office is dedicated to studies of concentration camps. Usually those who run concentration camps treat healthier people better and sicker people worse. When concern for human dignity and human life is absent, all that matters is the labor that can be extracted. Stalin's Gulag was run according to this logic of reverse health care. Because Soviet administrators regarded prisoners as economic units, health care was distributed according to calculations about productivity. Medical attention meant figuring out who could be exploited for longer and who should be discarded sooner. Stronger prisoners might be cared for so long as they were productive, but weaker ones were allowed to die, often released from the camp to perish beyond its gates—so as not to be counted, so as not to figure in the record.

If we think that the Gulag is the depth of horror, what then is the summit of good? Part of the answer is to recognize that all people have an equal right to health care, regardless of how productive or profitable they are judged to be. That is a conclusion that a number of wise people, including Americans, drew from the horrors of the twentieth century.

The idea that health care is a right can seem strange to Americans today. Yet officially the United States has been committed to such a right for more than seventy years. After Nazi Germany was defeated in the Second World War, and as the United States engaged the Soviet Union in a long Cold War, Americans helped to draft and Americans signed agreements that articulated a human right to health care.

The constitution of the World Health Organization, founded in 1946, states: "The enjoyment of the highest attainable standard of health is one of the fundamental rights of every human being without distinction of race, religion, political belief, economic or social condition." The Universal Declaration of Human Rights of 1948 states: "Everyone has the right to a standard of living adequate for the health and well-being of himself and of his family, including food, clothing, housing and medical care and necessary social services." Most nations' constitutions enshrine a right to health care. The list includes Japan and Germany, whose new constitutions the United States influenced after defeating them in the Second World War. Today Germans and Japanese live longer and healthier lives than Americans.

Americans helped to establish health care as a human right around the world. Why then is health care not seen as such in the United States? Why are Americans not protected by the agreements that our government signed? Should we accept that citizens of other democracies enjoy a right that we are denied, and live longer and healthier lives than we do? Many of us seem to find that acceptable. Why?

❀ ❀

I think that our death wish has to do with a growing imbalance between solitude and solidarity, with a rage that, when not balanced by empathy, undermines rather than affirms our freedom. When I think back to where I come from, and to the ways I was ill before my crisis, I get an inkling of one of the sources of this imbalance.

In my hospital diary I have a sketch of the house where my children were waiting for me, and a sketch of a barn in Ohio. I was born fifty-five years after my father's father, a farmer. I was a reasonably athletic kid, but my grandfather's forearms were twice as thick as mine. The veins stood out on his hands and up his arms. When he took my wrists in his hands, I could not move. He was missing a finger or two as a result of accidents with farm machinery, but this didn't seem to make a difference. My other grandfather, my mother's father, was also a farmer. Though he never talked about what he could make and repair, it was seemingly everything. He died on his tractor. Perhaps my grandfathers complained about pain during their working lives. But I can't imagine their doing so. No one ever told me directly not to talk about pain, but I took this in very young. When at the age of eight I greensticked my left wrist trying to stiff-arm an ancient oak on my father's wooden sled, I didn't make a sound (until I saw the x-ray).

A decade or so later, I sprained, or perhaps broke, my left ankle playing basketball on a playground in Washington, D.C. I taped the ankle up around a brace, lay low for a few days, and went to work with a cane for a summer. I didn't see any x-rays then, since I had neither money nor insurance. I broke the same ankle later, when I did have insurance, and got treatment. I broke seven ribs in my twenties and thirties: five on other people's elbows on the basketball court, two on my own elbow while falling in a Paris church complex known as the Valley of Grace. I dislocated a finger getting a rebound, and long ago stopped counting the broken toes. All this was before I broke my back and was diagnosed with osteoporosis. I am older now, but my bones have improved, thanks to some sensible medical advice.

I got my first migraine headache as a sophomore in college, after staying up all night working on a research project. By the time I went to England to study history in 1991, the migraines were regular. Ignoring this pain seemed not to work; it is impossible to get distance from one's own head. Before there were medicines that worked to halt migraines (triptans), I found myself in the emergency room every few weeks, everywhere I lived and worked, in Europe and America. Occasionally I passed out from the pain. Once there was medication I took it, and the frequency of visits to the emergency room decreased to once every few months.

When I got sick in December 2019, my diffidence about pain was unhelpful. The ache in my abdomen started during a business trip to Germany. I hailed a cab in Munich in the middle of the night and asked to be taken to a hospital. I failed to convey to the doctors there how much I hurt. I looked fine, did not complain much, was released. The German doctors thought that I had a viral infection and that my abdomen would hurt for a while.

When my appendix burst I did not realize what had happened and ignored the pain: after all, I had been told that I had an infection and that it would hurt for a while. I did the things in Germany that I was supposed to do, then flew to the United States with a perforated appendix. After a couple of days feeling fatigued at home, I went to the hospital and underwent an appendectomy. By then the burst appendix had seeded an infection in my liver, which was visible on the scans taken before the operation. The German doctors had seemingly overlooked my appendicitis; the American ones certainly neglected my liver infection; but somewhere in the mix is the difficulty I have in talking about physical pain.

My tolerance of pain comes from the same place as the rage that saved my life. It has helped me to do work that I value. Yet enduring pain in silence also creates a vulnerability, one that I think I share with other Americans. No one can endure extreme pain indefinitely. If there is a pill, we will all one day take the pill. If there is no one to talk to, no other form of medical care, we will keep taking the pill. The normality of enduring the pain then, imperceptibly, becomes the normality of taking the pill. What never changes is the lack of human contact. We can slip from silence about pain to silence about addiction, as millions of Americans have done.

In the hospital I was given oxycodone after three surgical procedures. I did not take it. Reading now the texts between my wife and the physician friend who was with me during my surgeries, I see an exchange sent after my skin and belly wall were punctured for my second and third liver drains:

"I'll try to talk to him again about taking the painkillers. He's always been wary of the opioids."

"Only if he wants to, Marci. I'm wary of the opioids too."

I am wary for a number of reasons. When I took them after breaking my back I felt like I was neither awake nor asleep and hated the sensation. My brother, a physicist who has had to undergo several surgeries, says that opioids are harder on his brain than the procedures and the anesthesia. Above all, when I see oxycodone I think of the bottles of it squirreled away in glove compartments, toolboxes, and under cushions all over Appalachia and the Midwest.

Over the decades wise doctors taught me that health care is more than pain and pills. In London in 1992, a doctor treating my migraines told me to "let people take care of you," which sounded strange to me at the time. In Paris, where I studied and lived alone for a year in 1994 and 1995, my migraines got so bad that I began to lose my sight. When I couldn't read my books and documents, or even distract myself by watching television, I realized that I had a problem. Stumbling to a hospital one night, unable to read the street signs or my map, I practiced my French for "feeling faint" and "seeing stars."

Later I saw a neurologist in Paris. I didn't have much money, but the fees were low. To get to his hospital I took a bus that went past the Eiffel Tower. I always gazed at it, and then at the Parisians on the bus, not a single one of whom even once spared it a glance. The neurologist, who examined me carefully and ran tests, suggested that my worsening condition had to do with separation from people I loved. As a young man,

I thought that he was either being very French or making fun of me. It took time for me to realize that he was onto something.

When I saw neurologists for my migraines in Europe in the 2000s and 2010s, after medication became available, I wanted them to just write me a prescription and let me go. Yet the European doctors liked to talk to me about the kind of life that I led, not just about the triggers of the migraines, but also about my priorities and practices. In Vienna, my internist sent me to a neurologist who really knows how to hunker down for a long chat. He made me laugh with his claim that he would find life not worth living if he had to avoid the things I couldn't eat and drink (namely schnitzel and wine). A few years ago, in an emergency room in Berlin late at night, I was befuddled when the doctor sat at my bedside for an hour talking about how I had spent my day. She gave me the medicine I wanted and a prescription that I could fill at a nearby all-night pharmacy, but she also wanted to think through with me how I became the person who visited hospitals in foreign countries at night.

The French, Austrians, and Germans have the same medicines we do—and they are less expensive and easier to get. In Germany I can get migraine medication without a prescription for a couple of euro at any pharmacy, even at an airport or railway station, provided that I take a moment to explain to the pharmacist why I need it. Every single part of that is impossible here. The difference is not that we have fancy chemicals and the Europeans do not. The difference is that doctors in Europe have time to do something beyond write out prescriptions. I have come to admire doctors who actually have a moment, want to think together with their patients, and seem to care. And I have come to realize that they are working within a system that enables and encourages all of that. And that such systems not only work better but also cost less than our own.

All of this care beyond our country, which I am very fortunate to have had, helps me to understand that there are alternatives beyond pills and pain. It is possible, if the appointments last longer than fifteen minutes and the doctors look at the person rather than the screen, for a patient's story to be told and understood. Medication is important, but it has its limits.

In the New Haven hospital on New Year's Eve, a nurse incorrectly administered my migraine medication, injecting it directly into my blood (intravenously) rather than into fatty tissue (subcutaneously). I felt like I had as a kid when I shocked myself on a wall socket, only this lasted longer. The mistake forced a rushed electrocardiogram. The incident reminded me that cardiac side effects are always a risk with triptans, and that my doctors had been trying to reduce my intake. Since leaving the hospital I have taken more seriously some of the good counsel about migraines that I have received over the years.

When there is no one with time to talk, no chance to find another approach, then we come to feel that we have to choose between pain and pills. In our country, where pharmaceutical advertisements are the main source of health information, we keep learning the lesson that suffering is our personal responsibility and that pills are the cure. When painkillers work, that creates a particular danger, because then we can ignore the deeper sources of suffering. We then get in trouble when we increase the dose, or find that medicine no longer works. Suffering and self-medicating are both lonely activities; they can feel like free choices, but they create an imbalance that leaves us in bondage.

American men slip from denying pain to denying

that they have a problem with painkillers. They slip from facing everything down, not taking the pill, to giving everything up, and just taking the pill. If life is lived between pain and pills, we end up with too much rage and not enough empathy, too much solitude and not enough solidarity.

The slope is steeper now than it was for my grandfathers' generation. Men of that age remembered the Great Depression and fought in the Second World War. To cheer up my kids during coronavirus isolation, one of their grandmothers sent a card about what her father had done in the Pacific campaign. Those were tougher times than these, was the message, and true enough. But the four decades after the war were an era of upward social mobility. The last four decades have been tough. The number of manufacturing jobs peaked in 1979. Factory jobs are not only rarer today, but also less likely to come with benefits and union cards. "Right to work" propaganda teaches Americans that we should go it alone, without unions, which leads to worse jobs, fewer friendships, more racism, poorer health care, and more anger.

Small farming is becoming untenable as a way of life. Farmers, the men who seemed invulnerable to me as a kid, now kill themselves in higher numbers than people in just about any other line of work. The federal suicide hotline for farmers has been eliminated. This is part of a broader demolition of the ramparts of the American dream. The welfare state, meant to complement the solitude of ambition with the solidarity of support, has been taken apart.

On farms and in factories, physical toughness had measurable payouts. Suffering was part of productivity. Facing things down could be the right thing to do. Until the 1980s, American fathers who worked hard could expect better life chances for their children. That is no longer true. When the economy changed and the welfare state weakened, when pain lost its purpose and suffering its efficacy, men were understandably confused. Americans perform less physical labor now and report more physical pain. Sadly, pain has become part of the economy, and of our political system. It used to be that American politicians competed with visions of a brighter future. Now a good deal of our politics is the solicitation and manipulation of pain.

Commercial medicine is part of the problem. The "pill mills" that emerged in the 1990s revealed the logical extreme of a medical system that offered a naked choice between suffering and pharmaceuticals. Pill mills are doctors' offices where physicians do nothing but prescribe opioids, usually in exchange for cash. The first one was seventy miles from my grandparents' farms, in Portsmouth, Ohio, which was a thriving manufacturing town when I was young. One year, the eighty thousand people of Scioto County, of which Portsmouth is the county seat, were prescribed ten million doses of opioids. Suffering was no longer productive for those who suffered, but it had become profitable for those who did not.

Opioids are a problem for women and men of all ages and backgrounds. White women in the South are living shorter lives, in part for this reason. The life expectancy of middle-aged white males has stagnated. Their American dream of solitary self-sacrifice has failed, and without the solidarity once offered by unions and the welfare state, they have been left alone with their resentment. If all we have is lonely rage, we fail, become addicted, listen to the wrong people, harm those we care about, and die. Opioids take over the mental space we need to contemplate, to think about children, spouses, friends, or anyone else.

The double desperation of pain and addiction affects our politics. People who lived in places wracked by opioids voted for Donald Trump. The one piece of information that best predicts whether Mr. Trump won or lost a county in November 2016 was the degree of opioid abuse. In Scioto County, ground zero of the opioid epidemic, Mr. Trump took a third more votes in 2016 than Mitt Romney had in 2012. It was a surprise when Donald Trump won Pennsylvania. He got the majority of votes in several Pennsylvania counties that Barack Obama had won four years before. Every single one of those counties was in public health crisis as a result of opioid abuse. This also held for the counties in Ohio that Barack Obama had won and Mr. Trump took four years later: all but one of them was in opioid crisis. Votes of desperation, like deaths of desperation, are understandable. Yet those who remain behind suffer. Desperate voters close off care to themselves, their families, and everyone else by voting for politicians who traffic in pain.

Solitude is salutary, up to a point. We are not free if we do not know how to be ourselves, by ourselves. Yet too much solitude makes freedom impossible, first for the lonely, and then for everyone else. A solitary rage is part of freedom, but only part. If we have no help from others, our rage no longer protects us but endangers everyone. Once pride becomes resentment, we forget that we need help and claim that only others do. A fury that lashes out blindly is no mark of liberty, but an opportunity for politicians who provide targets for the anger. The downward spiral from pain to desperation and from pride to resentment is something that politicians like Mr. Trump understand and accelerate. They want people staggered by suffering, and so they oppose health care. Pain is their politics; their propaganda is a death trap.

Such politicians tell white people that they are too proud and upstanding to need insurance and public health, which, they say, would only be exploited by others less deserving (blacks, immigrants, Muslims). Flattery lubricates the downward slide to death: white Americans are told to face pain as solitary individuals, and that they betray themselves and their country if they admit that they need support. Only dark-skinned whiners, goes the story, ask for help. Of course, the elected representatives who say such things have their own health care provided by the government, and are denying something to their constituents that they know works for them. But hypocrisy is the least of their sins. Flattering while denying care adds sadism to manslaughter.

Everyone is drawn into a politics of pain that leads to mass death. Opposing health care because you suspect it helps the undeserving is like pushing someone else off a cliff and then jumping yourself, thinking that your fall will be cushioned by the corpse of the person you murdered. It is like playing a round of Russian roulette in which you load one bullet in the cylinder of your revolver and two in the other fellow's. But how about not jumping off cliffs; how about not playing Russian roulette? How about we live and let live, and all live longer and better?

Between the choice to live in pain and the choice to take pills, there should be a world of alternatives: health care that we can find, or that can find us. This would mean easier access to doctors, but also to other, simpler means of health. A great deal of physical pain, for example, is best treated with physical therapy and physical exercise. These options require human contact, and do not generate the quick profits of pharmaceuticals and surgical implants. If we are concerned about American health, and American freedom, then everyone should be insured, and everyone's insurance should cover what helps to relieve pain. We need a system of solidarity that no individual can create but from which every individual would gain.

※ ※

It is easy to fall into mental habits that make the status quo seem acceptable. It is tempting to find meaning in suffering and death. In this way well-meaning Americans provide rationalizations for those in power who hurt and kill. When someone dies we can tell ourselves that it had to be so, that it happened for a reason, that it was God's will. These beliefs prevent us from challenging a system of commercial medicine that treats us as sources of profit rather than as children of God. My suffering only has meaning if I learn from it, and my death would have been senseless. I am unconvinced that God wants my fellow Americans to suffer and die so that commercial medicine can make a few people rich.

It is also tempting to rest on the laurels of tradition, to refer back to the eighteenth century, to say that the Founding Fathers did not imagine modern public health. There are many things, of course, that they did not imagine. It is impossible for me to believe, as a citizen and as a historian, that the Founding Fathers wanted an America where people would live shorter and worse lives than necessary, where the sickness of the many would become a zone of profit for the few. The optimism in the preamble of the Constitution rings down the centuries: good government means justice, tranquility, welfare, liberty. A common defense. If we take pride in our Constitution and know its purposes, we apply the aspirations of its authors to our own times.

Toughing things out and avoiding doctors might have made sense two hundred years ago. I was released from the hospital into the coronavirus pandemic, shelter-at-home, and remote learning with two kids in elementary school, and have been reading about the history of the Revolutionary era with my son. Together we learned that George Washington died after three doctors bled him four times; he would have been better off not calling for them. Benjamin Franklin once wrote to John Jay that he feared the medicine more than the malady, which at the time made sense. A quick way to rub the romance from the Revolutionary War is to learn how the wounded were treated. Nothing was understood about infection then, so doctors did not wash their hands or sterilize their cutting tools. Brutal amputations were common, pus and swelling were misunderstood as signs of healing rather than infection, and burns were treated by bleeding the patient. Life expectancy for colonists was about forty years, and for the Africans they enslaved much less. Diseases brought from Europe, such as smallpox, drastically shortened the lives of the continent's native peoples.

I find it inconceivable that the founders of this country, the men who valued justice, tranquility, and welfare, would have wished for us to relive their wretched moment in the history of medicine. Certainly they never said any such thing. Indeed, much of the sadness in their correspondence with one another concerns personal sickness, the illness of friends, and the plagues that wracked the cities of the young republic. It was impossible to summon Congress one year because of an epidemic of yellow fever, a disease that was not then understood. We now know that it is transmitted by mosquitoes, and have a vaccine. Benjamin Franklin, Thomas Jefferson, and their peers were interested in saving Americans from yellow fever, smallpox, and other diseases against which we now have vaccinations or treatments. Jefferson thought that health was the most important element of a good life, after morality.

Now that we have better knowledge of the natural world, we can consider health care as a human right. The Constitution does not prevent us from doing so. On the contrary: its authors had the wisdom to specify that "the enumeration in the Constitution, of certain rights, shall not be construed to deny or disparage others retained by the people." This leaves room for a right to health care. If we accept Jefferson's famous trio of rights to "life, liberty, and the pursuit of happiness," the case for a right to health care is made. If we have a right to life, we have a right to the means of living. If we have a right to pursue happiness, then we have a right to the care that allows us to do so. Without health, said Jefferson very sensibly, there is no happiness. The right to liberty implies a right to health care. We are not free when we are sick. And when we are in pain, or when we are anxious about illness to come, rulers seize upon our suffering, lie to us, and strip away our other freedoms.

LESSON 2.

Renewal begins with children.

In my hospital diary I have notes about what my children were doing in January. "Soccer practice harder." "Friends E and A over." "School starting." I was proud of my son and daughter for getting up in the morning and going to school when they knew what was wrong. When I was too sick for them to visit me, my wife told me about their days. My children also wrote me notes and drew me pictures, which I taped to the wall or folded up and kept in my diary. When I could move around, they started to visit me, one at a time. My daughter wanted hugs and gave me food. "Daddy," said my son, "I keep dreaming you die."

In the hospital, and then after I was released from the hospital, in my office, and then after pandemic shut me out of my office, I kept thinking of my children. The rage and the empathy I felt when I was sickest had to do with them; but even after these emotions slowly cleared, a tearing sensation remained. The enormity of what could have been their loss, my loss, our loss, was too great to hold within a few days. Even after school was closed and I saw them at home all day every day, the anguish kept radiating through my days and nights, expressed in anxious searches for them around the house, and in my dreams.

One night I woke from a nightmare to the realization that my photographs of their first few years of life were not backed up. I sat straight up and got out of bed. My dream had revealed to me a small remedy of my sense of separation; keeping the past recorded was a way of binding the children to me, one that I could manage in my weakened state. I found the old computer, rigged it up, got a hard drive, and went to work. As I backed up the photographs, each of them flitted over the screen in reverse chronological order, milliseconds and memories. They ended, or began, with images of my newborn son, tiny in a blue blanket and mittens.

❀ ❀

Those photographs were of my children, but the anguish I felt could have been felt by anyone. The beginning of life is particular to each parent and yet general to parenthood, an experience distinct from everything else in life, and yet shared across the planet. As those 14,810 images wound me backward through the last decade, I thought about the renewal of life that comes along with birth, and about what makes the passage easier, or harder. That blue blanket and those mittens belonged to a public hospital in Vienna, Austria, where my son was born. That hospital and that city certainly made things easier for us. That pregnancy and birth, the first for Marci and me, created a sense of what good health care felt like from the inside: intimate and inexpensive.

During all the months of obstetrical care in Vienna in 2009 and 2010 we paid almost nothing: small fees for doctor visits, on top of a modest monthly insurance premium. We were paying extra (although not much) to see a private doctor who had been recommended to us; we could have seen an obstetrician at no cost. Throughout the pregnancy (and after the birth) my wife carried a handy "mother-child passport," recognized throughout the country, where doctor visits, test results, and inoculations were recorded. Rather than looking at a screen when my wife entered the hospital or doctor's office, a nurse or physician would greet us and ask to see the "passport."

The city of Vienna offered us subsidized (and entertaining) birthing classes. Austrians usually speak a neutral version of German to foreigners, but in intimate settings switch to dialect, which is harder to understand. I found myself on a mat performing routines with balls and bells for reasons that were less than clear. But birthing class was fun and made the rhythm of pregnancy more social. Because the couples had all conceived at about the same time, we kept seeing familiar people in the same stages of pregnancy. We made friends whose children have grown up with ours.

At every step of the pregnancy, right through childbirth, we had the sense, even as foreigners, that the medical system was designed for the child and for us. There was never the creepy moment that one has inside American commercial medicine: when you wonder just why something was done or not done, or why some weird evasive phrase was just uttered, or why a doctor or nurse behaved oddly or slipped away. In the United States, one often has the feeling that there is a hidden logic dictating events, because there is: a logic of profit. In Austria, it was clear that the goal was the welfare of the unborn child. Prenatal visits were mandatory, in exchange for access to the welfare state.

The difference between a logic of profit and a logic of life can be seen in the timing. In the third trimester of pregnancy, women in Austria are instructed to come to the hospital if they are bleeding, if their water breaks, or if their contractions are twenty minutes apart. In the United States, expectant mothers are told to wait longer, until their contractions are three or four minutes apart. This is one reason why babies are born in back seats here, and why American mothers and newborns end up dead. In America the worry is that expectant mothers will arrive too early and occupy a hospital bed for too long; in Austria the system is designed to get them where they need to be in good time for a healthy birth.

On the evening that my wife went into labor in Vienna, we were immediately admitted into a clean, quiet room in the public hospital. We had to sign one piece of paper. We fretted that we had come too early, but there was no pressure to go back home. Marci's labor was long, difficult, and complicated, so we were glad to be in a hospital for the duration. After the birth, mother and baby were required to remain in the hospital for ninety-six hours. The idea was to ensure that newborns got a good start and that mothers learned how to breastfeed.

I was allowed to visit from nine in the morning until five in the afternoon, so I could see how this worked. Every day there were sessions for parents about how to bathe a baby and change a diaper. The nurses rotated through the ward, adjusting nipples and mouths, and giving instructions. The new mothers lacked the privacy that Americans might have expected, but they did have the unremitting attention of qualified people whose priority was their babies. The nurses were not interested in how the mothers felt about breastfeeding; they had a program to make sure that breastfeeding began. They knew what they were doing, and after four days the newborns and the mothers did as well. About ninety percent of mothers in Austria learn how to breastfeed. When we walked out, mother and baby were ready. We signed no forms and paid no bills.

During those birthing classes I had been the object of pity. Each session began with instruction for couples, during which my wife and I shared a mat and puzzled over Viennese slang for body parts. Then the men and women were divided and expected to talk amongst themselves about common concerns. I don't know what American men would talk about at such a moment; the Austrian dads talked about the freedom afforded to them by their welfare state. They had a choice among three parental leave options, all of which seemed impossibly generous to me. The other guys were making decisions about how *two years* of *paid* parental leave would be divided between the mother and father. I tried to tell my new friends that my wife and I had a relatively good deal, thanks to my university; they found one semester for one partner sadly inadequate. Their expressions turned to horror when I told them about the norm of parental leave in the United States. The idea that mothers might have twelve weeks but might have nothing, and that fathers expected nothing, seemed barbaric. They were right. It *is* barbaric. And it makes parents and children less free.

As they pointed out, and as I was ashamed to realize, my notion that three months of parental leave for one partner was generous depended wholly on my knowledge that what my wife had was better than what other Americans had. My own attitude was contributing to the general problem. My relative satisfaction with health care that was less terrible than others' kept me from seeing how disastrous the entire system was, and how much better it could be. Every American could and should have parental leave better than what my wife and I had. If Austria could do it, why not us? Every single citizen of Austria, regardless of status and wealth, had better choices than I did. I had been duped, like many Americans who have less-bad access to health care and public services. Everyone, my friends sensibly proposed, should have the same options, and those options should allow a family to make it through.

After our son was born, I wanted to have time with him and give his mother a bit of a break from us, and so took walks with him around Vienna between his feedings. I enjoyed pushing a stroller around the city. I'd like to think that I would have done this anyway, but it is important to acknowledge how policy changes practices, and how practices change norms. Thanks to parental leave, walking around with babies was a normal thing for men to be doing. It was nice to occasionally share a nod of acknowledgment with other guys: hey, what a great thing, we are dads. It was also nice to be treated kindly by the waitresses and waiters at the cafés where I would stop when my son slept.

Thanks to such encounters, my attitude to the German language began to change. The horrors of the twentieth century had made German a language of death. As old ladies on the sidewalk complimented me on my beautiful child, German became a language of life.

❧ ❧

The birth of our second child two years later in America was different.

Our son had been born without the artificial induction of labor and without a caesarean section. The obstetricians in the Vienna public hospital had been very patient during the labor, far more so than their American colleagues could have been. My wife turned forty during her second pregnancy, which triggered an American protocol for labor to be artificially induced by her due date. These protocols make little sense: it's not age as such that matters, but certain conditions that become more likely in women with age.

In large matters and small, machine protocols get between patients and their caretakers. The computer programs are about billing, and so fail to account for basic human needs. Doctors and nurses who get used to following protocols retrain themselves to ignore the actual patient. When I was in the hospital I noted some examples of this in my diary.

I took medications on a schedule. I wrote down the times and doses, partly because I had lost trust in the system, partly because I wanted to sleep at night. I was allowed to take acetaminophen every six hours for pain. I would ask the nurses not to wake me at night simply because six hours had passed. Sometimes this worked; sometimes it didn't. When I would skip a dose, I would try to explain that the schedule should reset, and that my next dose could be at any time, rather than six hours after the scheduled time for the dose that I had not taken. Sometimes nurses went along with me, sometimes with the screen. I might in the evening have three medications to take, one at 10:00, one at 11:00, and one at midnight. A savvy and motivated nurse would alter the timing of the doses during the day so that, after a couple of days of nudging, I could take all three pills at the same time and then go to sleep. Helping a patient sleep meant bucking the system, which is absurd. Another nurse, though, might insist that what the computer told her to do she had to do, and would wake me up to satisfy the algorithm.

In more significant cases, like a pregnancy, the cost of screen obedience can be much greater. When a computer program mindlessly flags "pregnant yes" and "40+ yes" and indicates that induction should take place by such and such a date, medical personnel find it easier to pacify the alert that pops onto the screen than to learn the story of a woman. Quietly, attention is turned to the algorithm—lifeless code that does not care—and away from the human who is hard at work creating another human. Although my wife was fit and the baby healthy, we were caught in this mechanical logic. We had to fight for the thirty extra minutes it took for labor to begin without induction. Happily, the second delivery was quicker and simpler than the first.

After the birth, the clock began to tick again, this time for our expulsion from the maternity ward. My wife was alone in a small room this time, without the buzz of mothers, babies, nurses, and fathers to which we had become accustomed in Vienna. Only with difficulty did she remember how to encourage a newborn to breastfeed; no one was around to help with that crucial part of the beginning of life. We did get a xerox with some schematic drawings of breasts and a phone number, but that is no substitute for an ever-present nurse who knows what to do. We also got a pile of paper and excessive bills. The phone number was for a lactation consultant, whom we did eventually see. In the United States one has to have good insurance or spare cash to see a lactation consultant, and most people do not. In this way, inequality affects the biology of babies from their first hours. It does no honor to the idea that "all men are created equal" to mandate an unequal start of life.

We have commercial medicine from cradle to grave because that is what we have chosen. There are better ways. When my wife and I left the hospital after my son's birth in Austria, we were given a kit with baby clothes and blankets in a handy diaper backpack. We also got a guide to all of the services the city of Vienna would offer, which included personal support for mothers who had trouble taking care of their babies, public child care, and public kindergartens and schools. All of these were free, provided parents took their children to the pediatrician and kept inoculation records in that "passport."

When we moved back to Austria with the children, aged one and three, we were stunned at the quality of the public preschool in our working-class neighborhood. It had the amenities and good cheer of the private day cares and preschools we had visited at home. And it was indeed entirely free of charge, aside from the forty euro a month that we were expected to contribute for the lunches (the local sourcing of which was a point of pride—and the subject of an hour-long parent-teacher meeting, not to mention an evening with the chefs).

Our three-year-old son was in a group of children aged three to six, and a bigger girl looked after him. His teacher made sure that he got the help that he needed in his new environment. We felt a little guilty about the trouble he caused, as the youngest child in the class, unsocialized in Austrian ideas of order. He would toddle over and knock down, with gusto, the complicated structures of blocks built by the bigger boys. We felt bad about that. There was a twinkle in his teacher's eye when we raised the subject: "But what a great feeling it is," she said kindly, "to knock something down."

When our son's kindergarten teacher realized that we would be taking him back to the United States after the school year, she wept in front of us.

❦ ❦

Each time our family lived in Austria I had some adjusting to do when we came back to America. I had trouble understanding why American parents were so feverishly engaged with their own children, yet so hesitant about making contact with other children.

In music class in New Haven, when my son was one or two, the children often refused to sit in front of their own caregivers in a ring. They preferred to crawl or toddle across the circle to another child or parent. I was always happy if a kid showed up: after all, what difference did it make where on the carpet they banged their drumsticks? And yet uncontrolled crawling or toddling always brought drama. Caregivers felt that their children should be right in front of them at all times: and so a tambourine-shaking hour was passed in the absurdity of adults springing up from faux-comfortable cross-legged sitting positions to hasten after wayward offspring. One little boy tended to hustle over to my son and me. I thought it was nice that he recognized us. One week his mother snarled at me: "What are you, the magnet of eighteen-month-olds?"

I was startled. Wasn't it nice when children smiled at adults and adults smiled back? Wouldn't it be good for the little boy to have some friendly exchanges with people beyond his own family? Wasn't socialization the point of getting out of the house and going to toddler music class? A few months into music class, I was speaking with another mother, with whom I had become friendly, about the tension. I asked her why the mothers seemed nervous when their children weren't right in front of them. Her answer gave me a lot to think about: "I guess it's because we know that at the end of the day we are doing this alone."

Imagine an America where mothers (and fathers, and other caregivers) did not feel that way. In Vienna my wife and I never did. People made way for the stroller and held open doors without being asked. I remember one morning when I was jogging down a hill, with my daughter in the stroller and my son standing on the board attached to its back, trying to catch the last subway train (at an aboveground stop) that would get the kids to kindergarten on time. The sun behind me, I could watch through the subway car's window as passengers pushed the button to open the doors for us, and then made way so that we could squeeze in.

This attitude to parents and young children is certainly not a result of Austrians being friendlier than Americans. It has to do with an understanding that rearing children is not something that a parent or even a family can do without help. The institutions that helped us, from the public hospital to the public kindergarten to the public transport (with an elevator at every subway stop), were not one-way gifts to families with children. They were an infrastructure of solidarity that held people together, making them feel that at the end of the day they were not alone.

※ ※

In America, birth is where our story about freedom dies. We never talk about how bringing new life into the world makes heroic individualism impossible. I certainly needed a great deal of help to be anything like a free person as a parent of young children, and I was not the one who had to bear and breastfeed the child, and had every possible advantage as a father. We are also silent about what we need to do to ensure, from the beginning, that children can lead lives that are as free as possible. We imagine freedom as an absence of restraints, and that is surely an important element of liberty. Yet the beginning of life shows us that it is also inadequate. A newborn left alone and unrestrained is not free. For children the contribution of others to freedom is even more significant than it is for parents.

How children are treated when they are very young profoundly affects how they will live the rest of their lives. That is perhaps the most important thing that scientists have to teach us about health and freedom today. In the nineteenth century, scientists explained how diseases spread, introducing a kind of factuality useful for longer, freer lives. In the late twentieth century, another group of scientists came to understand the importance of early childhood for the rest of life. It takes courage for adults to grasp this, because it means that caring about freedom means caring about children. But if we do, we can begin a renewal of a land of the free.

The capacities that people need in order to operate as free adults develop when we are small. The skills that we will apply to become unique human beings are created during the first five years of life, as the brain grows to nearly its full size. As infants and toddlers interact with other people, will and speech and thought emerge. We learn as very small children, if we ever learn, to recover from disappointment and to delay pleasure. Abundant research shows what allows these capacities to develop: relationships, play, and choices.

To be free involves having a sense of one's own interests and of what one needs to fulfill them. Thinking about the constraints of life under pressure requires an ability to experience, name, and regulate emotions. Freedom has to do with choice, but we can only choose among options we see. When we are trapped in fear we see everything in binary terms: us or them, fight or flight. Children who learn to name and regulate their emotions have a greater chance of opening up space for positive feelings, even at moments of stress. Without those positive emotions we are less free, because we cannot see the various escapes and innovations that we might need at a moment of danger, or use to thrive and prosper at better times.

The paradox of freedom is that no one is free without help. Freedom might be solitary, but freedom requires solidarity. An adult who has learned to be free in solitude benefited from solidarity as a child. Freedom is thus a loan paid out and paid back over generations. Children need intense and thoughtful attention during those first five years. This special time cannot be given by children to children, nor by adults to adults. Children can only borrow this special kind of time from adults. They can pay back the loan only later, when they themselves are grown, to the children who are yet to come. A free country thrives over generations.

As anyone who has tried to raise children in America knows, time is very hard to come by. It is easy to say that children need trusting relationships, unstructured play, and activities that encourage choices. Say it out loud to an American parent and expect a patient smile, in the best case. How is this time to be found when parents work? We know the answer. Mothers should have four days in maternity wards after birth, as a matter of law. Both parents need substantial maternity or paternity leave, predictable scheduling at work, paid sick days, public childcare, and paid vacations. These things are normal elsewhere and possible here.

Mothers and families also need calm during life's difficult passages, of which the bearing and rearing of children is one. Families who can count on good public schools for their children and reliable pensions for themselves will be less anxious about life and more available for their young children. If parents and caretakers know that they and their children have a right to health care, they will have more of the time and patience that they need to help their children become free.

LESSON 3.

The truth will set us free.

After my appendectomy on December 15th, 2019, I found myself identifying with others in a strangely intense way. Although no one had told me so, my liver was infected. Weakness brought me closer to people, made me more open to their stories. I paid attention to things I might have overlooked, like the words in front of churches as Christmas drew near. An announcement board in downtown New Haven asked whether "this Christmas we mean to celebrate one migrant family and separate, detain and deport the rest." That summoned the story of Mary and Joseph and the difficult journey of a pregnant woman who gave birth far from home. The comparison of their plight to that of the undocumented migrants in nearby detention centers hit me harder than I would have expected.

The surgeon who had performed my appendectomy told me that it was safe to travel, so I went to Florida to join my extended family for a long-planned Christmas vacation. The idea was that I would recuperate on the beach. Matters took a different turn. I was hospitalized in Florida on the morning of December 23rd after my limbs began to tingle, but was discharged the next day with no diagnosis. I fell into a malaise on Christmas Day that worsened on the twenty-sixth and twenty-seventh. I began to lightly hallucinate, recognizing people I knew in the faces of strangers. Passersby began to resemble my brothers. My wife, Marci, got me and our children back to Connecticut on the night of December 28th. It was an unpleasant flight.

After those seventeen hours in the emergency room of a New Haven hospital in that yellow-curtained alcove on December 29th, and after a procedure on my liver, I was admitted to the room where I spent the last days of the year and the first days of the new one raging and contemplating. I shared that room with a Chinese man who was suffering from a number of afflictions. He spoke two words of English when I arrived and four when I left, and so doctors and nurses communicated with him through a translation service or with the help of his family. This meant that a great deal of personal and medical information was communicated loudly, slowly, and repeatedly.

I came to understand that my neighbor was fourteen years older than I, that he worked as a busboy, that he spoke Cantonese rather than Mandarin, and that he was in withdrawal from nicotine and alcohol after five decades of daily smoking and drinking. That last fact made me all the more appreciative of his friendly demeanor and gracious attitude. When he saw me taking walks, he realized that he could do the same, and always smiled in greeting when we crossed paths in the hallway. He wore headphones when he watched television and tried not to awaken me when I slept.

My roommate arrived on New Year's Day, not long after returning from China, the day after authorities in that country confirmed the existence of a novel coronavirus. I soon developed a mysterious respiratory problem. I could not inhale deeply, and found it difficult to talk. My friends and family were troubled that I could speak by telephone for only a few minutes without seeming weary and losing my voice. Scans showed that both of my lungs had partially collapsed. At the time, doctors suggested that my right lung was compressed by the liver inflammation. But my scans actually revealed that my left lung had collapsed more severely than my right.

Like me, my roommate had respiratory issues but got over them, and was in the hospital for other reasons. Sharing close quarters with him, I couldn't help but observe how he was treated and how his symptoms were evaluated. I was drawn into his story. Blood tests pointed in a number of directions. A parasite from raw fish eaten during his visit to China seemed the likely culprit. When cancer was ruled out, it was my first happy moment in the hospital. When I was discharged I gave him my good wishes through a friend who wrote them as a text message in Mandarin; he wrote a very kind response and had his phone translate it for me. "You too please take care of yourself well."

❦ ❦

My roommate was an example of two ways medicine can get to truth. Sometimes treatment is a matter of thinking along with the patient, focusing on a story, and making sense of it. I could hear his story coming together for the doctors, who perhaps paid more attention and remembered better as a result of the effort it took to communicate. Sometimes medicine is a matter of tests, a search for information by experimental means. This, too, was important for my neighbor. Although the doctors and nurses could not communicate with him directly, they did know which tests to run for which symptoms, and how to interpret the results. Within the limits of their clinical knowledge and the available tests, they could pin down what he did and did not have.

In early 2020, our federal government failed us in both ways. There was no sensible discussion of the history of pandemics, and no procedure to test for the new plague. In January, it failed to do what was so obviously necessary: acquire a test for the new coronavirus and apply it on a massive scale in the United States. The president's administration had disbanded the sections of the National Security Council and the Department of Homeland Security meant to deal with epidemics, as well as a special unit in the Agency for International Development that was meant to predict them. American health experts had been withdrawn from the rest of the world. The last officer of the Centers for Disease Control and Prevention assigned to China was called back to the United States in July 2019, a few months before the epidemic began.

The president had overseen budget cuts for institutions responsible for public health, and in early 2020 announced his intention to cut them again. As the year began, Americans were denied the basic knowledge they needed to make decisions on their own, or to press their government to take action. On February 1st, the surgeon general of the United States tweeted "Roses are red / Violets are blue / Risk is low for #coronavirus / But high for the flu." Since we were not testing, he had no idea what he was talking about.

In January and February 2020, the novel coronavirus spread silently through the country. During those two essential months, when the mathematics of contagion demanded an urgent response, and when testing and contact tracing could have contained the epidemic, we did less than nothing. Mr. Trump praised himself while ignoring the warnings he was given. On January 24th, he praised China for its response to the coronavirus: "China has been working very hard to contain the Coronavirus. The United States greatly appreciates their efforts and transparency. It will all work out well. In particular, on behalf of the American People, I want to thank President Xi!" On February 7th, he renewed his praise: "Great discipline is taking place in China, as President Xi strongly leads what will be a very successful operation."

When Americans known to be infected were evacuated from a cruise ship in February, they were flown back to the United States on an airplane with hundreds of other people who were not yet infected. The people infected en route then scattered freely throughout the country. This indefensible sloppiness by the federal government guaranteed that the disease would spread. As February came to an end, Mr. Trump spoke of a "miracle" that would save us: "It's going to disappear. One day it's like a miracle, it will disappear."

The secretary of commerce predicted that the virus would bring jobs to the United States, while his department arranged for American manufacturers to sell protective medical masks to China. In fact, tens of millions of jobs disappeared, American unemployment rates reached highs not seen since the Great Depression, and shortages of masks cost American lives. On February 24th, Mr. Trump insisted that the coronavirus was "under control." This was not true. In early March he said that anyone who wanted a test could get tested. That was a lie. By the end of February, the United States had tested only three hundred and fifty-two people, about as many as the graduating senior class in the high school down the block from my house. South Korea had by then tested seventy-five thousand people.

The time lost in stupefaction and mendacity, the first two months of 2020, could never be regained. By the end of April, South Korea was down to fewer than ten new cases a day, while the United States had more than twenty-five thousand new cases a day. At the end of April *twice* as many people had died in the Connecticut county where I am recuperating (population less than one million) than in the entire country of South Korea (population fifty-two million). By the end of May *three times* as many people had died in New Haven County than in all of South Korea. This was no fluke. The seven American *counties* with the most covid deaths would now rank among the top twenty *countries*. These are the simple truths.

Since the truth sets you free, the people who oppress you resist the truth. In any catastrophe, especially one of their own making, tyrants will find a mixture of blaming others and excusing themselves that includes an enticing element of what we want to hear. In early 2020, people naturally wanted to hear that there was no coronavirus in the United States. But we cannot be free and deluded. History remembers the British prime minister Neville Chamberlain unkindly because he told his people what they wanted to hear in 1938: that there need be no war. History remembers Winston Churchill kindly because he told the British what they needed to hear: that Hitler had to be stopped.

Before I got sick I was reading *The Lord of the Rings* to my son and daughter. A noble character in Tolkien's saga, the wizard Gandalf, is a teller of unwanted truths. He has great powers, but cannot save the world by himself. His task is to build a coalition by convincing others of the reality of a threat. Time after time, Gandalf is ignored by the less wise, scorned as a bearer of bad news. In the story, as in life, people choose ignorance to supply themselves with an excuse for submission: how could we have known, what could we have done? This is one way to be human, but it is no way to be free. Gandalf finally retorts that without knowledge freedom has no chance. People lose life and liberty if they cannot identify a threat and make preparations. Not wanting to know means asking for oppression. Not wanting to know about disease means asking politicians to surveil your body, and to manipulate you with the emotions that accompany mass death.

The truth takes work. Facts do not often line up with what we believe, want to believe, or are led to believe. Facts are what we apprehend when we place ourselves at the right distance between our emotions and the world around us. Getting to the facts always requires some labor, work that the people at the top of the federal government chose not to do. It would have taken just a bit of effort, and just a bit of courage, to admit that there was a problem, and to organize tests and tracing. Since these were lacking, a hundred and fifty thousand Americans died needlessly.

❦

A test for a disease reflects knowledge of a microbe and of our bodies. When we test we extend factuality into the world, one person at a time. The knowledge that arises from a test is about you and the world. It is shared: you know what the test takers know. Had we tested Americans in early 2020, we would have spread factuality into our country, and given doctors and everyone else a sense of what to do.

Mr. Trump proclaimed that he understood the mysteries of the world, promised Americans a miracle, and hawked eye of newt. He promoted hydroxychloroquine without basis; it was associated with higher death rates in patients, and seems to have killed a number of veterans to whom it was administered. A federal official who quite properly questioned the allocation of taxpayer money to it was fired. Another who reported shortages in needed equipment was also fired. This is how tyranny works: the truth tellers are banished as the sycophants huddle close. Mr. Trump then wondered aloud whether Americans should inject themselves with disinfectants.

We did not test for coronavirus for a reason that has been understood for thousands of years, at least since Plato. No one likes bad news; an unchecked ruler never hears what he should from his yes-men; he then projects fictions, which he may actually believe, upon everyone else. This leads to suffering and death, which means more bad news, and so the cycle starts again. Once Mr. Trump made it clear that his priority was to see low counts of infected Americans, the simplest way to please the tyrant was not to count. On March 6th, Mr. Trump said that he preferred to leave infected Americans on a cruise ship because "I would rather—because I like the numbers being where they are—I don't need to have the numbers double because of one ship that wasn't our fault." Two months and tens of thousands of needless deaths later, Mr. Trump still evinced the same attitude: "by doing all this testing, we make ourselves look bad." On June 15th, Mr. Trump proclaimed, "If we stop testing right now, we'd have very few cases, if any." Five days later he praised himself for an order to "slow the testing down."

Such magical thinking was tyrannical, delusive, and irresponsible. It was tyrannical, in Plato's sense of the word, because it revealed the tyrant's narcissistic concern for his own image ("the numbers") over the reality lived by others—in this case the reality of an epidemic that would kill more Americans than any in the past hundred years. It was delusive because it confused looking away with taking action, the absence of testing with the absence of infection. Mr. Trump's unwillingness to test did not mean that we were healthy, only that we were ignorant. It was irresponsible because it transferred accountability for American lives away from himself and our government. As Mr. Trump denied any "fault," the disease was spreading in our country, unobserved and untreated. His focus on a foreign source of "fault" meant that no one here was to blame. When no one bears responsibility, no one has to do anything.

Historians know that before we understood disease we blamed it on others, often people we had treated badly. In the fourteenth century, Christians used the bubonic plague as an excuse to murder Jews to whom they owed money. In the fifteenth and sixteenth centuries, European sailors transmitted a number of new diseases to the New World and brought one back. Syphilis came first in the bodies of Spanish sailors, and so the English at first called it "Spanish." Italians called it "French," as did Shakespeare. The Poles called it "German" or "American." Russians called it "Polish." In the Ottoman Empire it was called "Christian."

After contagion was understood, some people mischaracterized the science by associating whole groups with bacteria and viruses, or by claiming that hidden enemies delivered biological weapons. American racists portrayed blacks as vessels of germs. The Nazis blamed venereal disease, typhus, and tuberculosis on Jews. Stalinists blamed pestilence on Americans, and Russians later said the same about AIDS. Russia claimed that coronavirus was an American bioweapon as early as January 2020. China soon said the same, while some American politicians blamed a Chinese bioweapons lab. The Republican Party, recognizing that Mr. Trump's coronavirus policy was catastrophic, planned its fall 2020 election campaigns around blaming China for everything.

Seeing disease as foreign obscures an essential fact: no matter where a contagion starts, we are all essentially the same in our vulnerabilities, and thus in our responsibilities. Scapegoating another group aligns our minds with authoritarianism. First, we believe a tyrant who tells us that we are immune because we are innocent and superior; then, when we get sick, we believe that we must have been unfairly attacked by someone else, since we are innocent and superior. The tyrant who lied to us about our immunity and superiority then tries to gather power from our suffering and resentment. When Mr. Trump invokes an "Invisible Enemy" when closing borders, or refers to the coronavirus as "Chinese," he takes part in a tradition that confuses and kills.

China does bear responsibility for ignoring the reality of the outbreak. Yet American policy was to repeat China's mistakes, after China had made them, and for a far longer time. For that only Americans can be blamed.

❦ ❦

Thomas Jefferson, Benjamin Franklin, and other men who founded this country were participants in the Enlightenment, an eighteenth-century expression of confidence that human life could be understood through the study of nature. A motto of the Enlightenment was "dare to know." Some of the most valiant people who followed that motto were the men and women of the nineteenth century who overturned folk wisdom and explained the principles of contagion. Their breakthroughs led to public hygiene and mandatory vaccination, two developments that are largely responsible for the extension of human life in the twentieth century.

Unfortunately, enlightenment can be undone. The fact that we can all be infected, and the consequence that we should all be checked, take courage to face. Mr. Trump lacked courage, and too many of us followed his lead. Knowledge about the world (for example, the number, location, and identity of infected people) can help us to manage the world's ruthlessness (for example, an exponential rate of infection). If we do not accept that we are part of nature, we cannot govern and we cannot live. Untested people were more likely to die, and more likely to spread the disease so that others died. Governors and mayors deprived of basic data about their constituents made decisions too late.

Once politicians embrace ignorance and death, their next move is to bluster and blame. Journalists who ask the right questions and local leaders who act to save lives must be ostracized, because they reveal authoritarians as cowards. Politicians who summon mass death with their own actions, as Mr. Trump did, will present it as inevitable, not their fault, the work of enemies, and then apportion the dying in a way that suits them. Death, and the fear of death, become political resources. Rather than extending health care to all, a tyrant will watch people die, and try to stay in power by riding the roiling emotions of the survivors. In America, the people who died first and fastest were African Americans, who as a rule did not vote for Mr. Trump.

A tyrant sees malady as opportunity, presenting himself as the rightful arbiter of life and death. Mr.

Trump made it clear that resources purchased with taxpayers' money would be distributed according to governors' loyalty to him. The federal government retreated from the massacre it had caused, telling the states to fight it out amongst themselves for medical resources. This needless competition drove up the prices of medical equipment and safety gear, making matters worse. Governors who tried to save lives were called disloyal. African Americans kept dying at catastrophic rates.

The Department of Justice requested the authority to detain any American without trial; meanwhile, it dropped charges against a man close to the president who had already pleaded guilty. Mr. Trump fired inspectors general across the federal government under cover of the pandemic, placing the rule of law in question and inviting corruption into the very center of public life. In April 2020, the pandemic was used to suppress votes in Wisconsin. An election that might have been delayed was forced, after decisions of the state and federal supreme courts, to take place with the vast majority of urban polling stations closed. This cast a shadow on elections to follow. Mr. Trump opined that the problem with unimpeded voting is that "you'd never have a Republican elected in this country again." He decried voting by mail, although he himself votes by mail. In April, Mr. Trump encouraged Americans to violently overthrow ("liberate") their state governments. In May, an African American named George Floyd, who had suffered from coronavirus and lost his job during the epidemic, was killed by a Minneapolis policeman. In the worst tradition of tyrants, Mr. Trump threatened military intervention to halt the protests that followed.

Our failure during a public health crisis is a sign of how far our democracy has declined. As we have hastened along the road to authoritarianism during the Trump administration, we have placed not only our liberties but our lives at risk. Democracies where law is respected and the press is robust respond better to pandemics than do authoritarian regimes. The combination of free speaking and free voting allows citizens to report what their rulers are doing, and to replace the ones who lie about matters of life and death. When democracy is limited, citizens die. One of the limits on our democracy is the vast and unregulated presence of money in politics, which means that in times of crisis private equity firms and insurance companies get more of a voice in matters of life and death than patients and doctors.

Around the world, authoritarian leaders lied about the severity of a plague, claimed their own countries were immune, punished the journalists who got it right, and then used the crises they created to consolidate power. Mr. Trump's behaviors followed the authoritarian pattern: a denial of reality, the claim of magical immunity, the harassment of reporters, the transformation of a problem he caused into a loyalty test for others, the cultivation of fear as a political resource. Authoritarians will allow people to die uncounted rather than admit that the number of dead in their country was high.

In the United States, we have both the highest death toll from coronavirus in the world (authoritarian disregard for life) and the certainty that it is a severe undercount (authoritarian resistance to facts). We know that that the official American death count is far too low, since people were dying when almost no testing was being done; since people continue to die throughout the country, at home and in hospitals, without being tested; since little counting of cases or deaths was done in nursing homes; since Florida has suppressed data about the number of deaths; and since there are large numbers of unexplained excess deaths every month.

In the end, authoritarians have little incentive to halt a pandemic, since they can thrive in an atmosphere of manipulated fear. The idea seems to be not to count Republicans who die, nor Democrats who vote. Democracy is needed for public health, but a public health crisis in a weak democracy like our own can be used to bring it down. Under the cover of pandemic, voting has been made more difficult. During mass demonstrations against racism, Mr. Trump has called for violence and domination. If fewer people vote in November 2020 this will be a crisis not only for democracy, but also for public health. If lies about illness lead to authoritarianism, we can expect more illness and more lies.

❦ ❦

If we need the truth to set us free, can the internet liberate us? We have been told that big data would rationalize our political decisions. Silicon Valley did nothing to help Americans in January and February 2020. That was a time, it might have seemed, when some rapid data crunching could have saved lives and the economy. That didn't happen, because big data is not the same thing as the knowledge humans need to thrive. Values such as life, health, and freedom do not matter to machines. Our staggering computer power brought us very little.

The people who ran the data companies understood the mathematics of contagion and sent their own employees home. But on the day that they did so, did they advise others to do the same? Did your feed ever remind you to wash your hands and to clean your phone? It did not, because doing those things would interrupt your session. The business model of social media companies is to keep eyeballs on screens and hands on touchpads so that emotions can be tracked for advertisers. The human body is most trackable when inert. The internet age is the age of obesity; a third of Americans are obese, and obese Americans are most at risk of dying from the coronavirus.

The word *data* does not mean what it used to. Now it means the things that we don't know. Social media companies know about you, but you do not know about them—nor do you know what they know about you, nor do you know how they learned it, or what they intend to do with it. Big data is generally about how your mind can be manipulated for profit, rather than how your body might better move through the world. It can reveal our particular cravings and fears, but not our common needs.

For that reason, big data did not tell us what we should have acquired in early 2020: tens of millions of tests, and a large stockpile of protective gear and ventilators. Big data was admittedly good at establishing which people wanted to hoard which thing and putting them in touch with Chinese vendors. When life was at stake during the coronavirus outbreak, big data could not discern whether an individual was infected. Only the testing of humans by humans gives us the knowledge that we need. The facts we need are about one body at a time. We get them only if we believe in the science and care enough to work together. No machine can do this work for us.

No social platform can improve health, since any algorithm with such a goal would alert people to shut down their computers, wash their hands, and get some exercise. No social platform can promote freedom, since social platforms aim at addiction. No social platform can promote truth, because truth, as Euripides realized twenty-five hundred years ago, is about human daring. We care about free speech not because a machine can dump endless garbage into the maw of our worst instincts, but because an individual human being can say something true that others do not know and that power wants hidden.

❦ ❦

Reporters are the heroes of our time; and like all heroes at all times they are too few. What we always need in a democracy, and what we needed desperately in early 2020, was not invisible big data but visible small facts: local news, reported by local people for local people, for the betterment of all. One reason why the novel coronavirus spread silently across America is that our country lacked the early warning system that we once took for granted: reporters who could have noticed new illnesses in their communities.

Reporting, like medical testing, is a way to produce facts. The reporter aims to be objective, getting close to an event while keeping emotions at a distance. A local newspaper conveys a sense of a shared world; the knowledge gained is credible. Like medical testing, reporting can tell us the things that we need to hear.

Freedom of speech becomes meaningful when we have something to talk about.

Journalists saved American lives in early 2020 by forcing an unwilling president to confront, if fitfully and belatedly, the reality of the coronavirus. Fatally, many Americans saw the confrontation between Mr. Trump's witchcraft and reporters' fact-checking as a partisan disagreement. Coronavirus seemed abstract because Americans had little or no local information about it. Since people did not know that the virus was already loose in their communities, that hospitals were already dealing with unexpected respiratory ailments, that nursing homes were already piling up bodies, the conversation in the White House seemed to be about politics rather than health, ideology rather than epidemiology.

Coronavirus was a local news story that could not be adequately covered because we lack the local reporters. Most American counties no longer have a proper newspaper. First, media was centralized in larger groups. Then the financial crisis of 2007–08 destroyed the livelihood of many reporters. Since then, the rise of social media has just about finished the job. Facebook and Google take the advertising revenue that newspapers once shared, though Facebook and Google do not report news.

Where social media has extinguished local journalism, distrust and ignorance reign. It is not simply that the facts are absent; it is that social media spread wild falsehoods, including about the pandemic, that never would have passed muster in a newspaper. The work of reporters affirmed the values of truth and well-being, and so helped to create trust. As local journalism fades, American attention shifts to national stories, ideology, and conspiracy theories designed to do harm.

Most of our country is now a news desert. News deserts kill us by depriving us of the information we need in our daily lives, and by leaving us confused at crucial moments when we need to act to protect our health and freedom. A familiar example is pollution. In the absence of local reporters, no one checks for unseemly relationships between politicians and companies. Projects that pollute the water or air simply PR their way into existence. If there are no local reporters, no one follows up on health complaints, or tests the water and air.

In Kentucky, the Louisville *Courier Journal* once forced action on strip-mining, pollution in the Ohio

River, and the dumping of sewage sludge and radioactive waste. Now that no reporter there (or anywhere in the state) has an environmental beat, these practices go unchecked. No one will cover continuing threats such as overlogging, mountain-topping, or the hazards of abandoned mines. Future dangers will emerge, go unreported, and kill people.

The coronavirus was used by the Trump administration as an excuse to legalize pollution, even though pollution makes it more likely that people will die from the coronavirus. We lack the reporters to cover the consequences.

A second example of how news deserts kill is the opioid crisis, which coincided with the collapse of local news. Americans in places like eastern Kentucky, western Pennsylvania, West Virginia, and southern Ohio knew, long before opioids made headlines, that something ominous had people in its grip. Years before major media covered it, opioid abuse was like cancer: a subject one didn't bring up at dinner because it probably concerned someone at the table. With too few local reporters writing about overdose, it took a decade for a national picture of the disaster to emerge.

The belated steps taken to address the opioid problem are now endangered by the spread of the novel coronavirus, which makes research and treatment much more difficult. By inviting a new epidemic we have extended a previous one.

In 2020, the lack of local reporters had the same consequence for the coronavirus as it had for pollution and opioids. We were missing the people whose work would have clarified a national disaster. We still do not know which communities were hit first. Months into the pandemic, millions of Americans were still reacting to hints and winks from Washington, because they had no local reporters to tell them that the illness was already infecting their neighbors. Conspiracy theories spread because social media had taken the place of local newspapers. Propaganda from Russia or China had easier access to dinner table conversation than realities down the block.

It was local reporters who provided the portraits of those who died. It was they who wrote about the mass dying in nursing homes. Local reporters found some of the places where bodies had been abandoned, and recorded some of the names of nurses and doctors who died. They revealed some of the occasions when states suppressed data about death. We can be sure, sadly, that most such stories were missed, simply because there were not enough journalists to cover them.

※ ※

Adam Mickiewicz, a great Romantic poet, began a famous poem with the lines:

Lithuania! My fatherland! You are like health.
Only he who has lost you can know your true worth.

Health is indeed like that; you appreciate it when it goes away. Truth is like health: we miss it when it fades. We can see the importance of medical knowledge and local knowledge now that they are dissipating.

If you lose your health completely, if you die, even the longing for health is gone. Something similar holds for truth. As we lose the people who produce facts, we are in danger of losing the very idea of truth. The death of truth brings the death of people, since health depends upon knowledge. The death of truth also brings the death of democracy, since the people can rule only when they have the facts they need to defend themselves from power. More than a hundred and fifty thousand of us died needlessly because all Americans were denied the truth. We now need the truth about what has happened, so that such things will not happen again.

We cannot be free without health, and we cannot be healthy without knowledge. We cannot generate this knowledge by ourselves as individuals: we need a general belief in the value of truth, professionals whose job is to produce facts, and robust institutions that support them. This is an example of the paradox of liberty: we cannot be ourselves without help; we cannot thrive in solitude without the solidarity of others. We can only balance solitude with solidarity when we share a factual world that enables us to see the larger meaning of our actions. During a pandemic we can choose solitude because we have solidarity with others whom we wish to see live and thrive. Local reporters warn us about dangers, help us to see challenges, and shield us from the divisive abstractions of ideology and the addictive emotions of technology.

As I write, we still need much, much more testing for the coronavirus. For the future, we need a sustained policy of supporting independent local reporting. A restoration of truth, and the application of truth to health, can begin as a reaction to a pandemic. We should have bailed out local newspapers in 2009; we should have bailed them out in 2020. They can be renewed now by a tax on the social media that exploited their labor and destroyed their livelihood, leaving the country poorer in spirit and weaker in health.

Yet the commitment to truth must go beyond the reflex to ward off mass death. We also need to remind ourselves what we know about leading a healthy life. Our present system of commercial medicine is poor at teaching us the basics. The centralization of traditional media in our country eventually imploded into the black hole of social media, which consumes factuality without producing it. Similarly, the centralization of commercial medicine weakens the voices of doctors, slowly turning them into mouthpieces for companies that own hospitals or sell drugs. What doctors know becomes harder and harder to hear, until at last it is crowded out by what makes money.

Doctors have their own methods of reaching truth: by scientific tests, but also through dialogue with patients. They can help us to restore the factual world, but only if we treat them with the respect they deserve.

LESSON 4.

Doctors should be in charge.

Now that I am a parent, and my parents are grand-parents, I think more about what I learned from them during childhood, during what my mother calls the "blur" of the 1970s. The time that she and my father spent with my two brothers and me during our early years still matters, every day, decades on. I try to appreciate this, and to recall some specific episode with them on their birthdays. I missed my mother's most recent birthday, though, because I was in a hospital in Florida.

During the two days and a night I spent there, from my mother's birthday into Christmas Eve, I was too anxious to sleep. My hands and feet were tingling and hot. I had been run through numerous tests during the day, but no doctors were around to talk about the results. So I looked out the window. I watched the moon appear in the sky, and stared at it through the night. The drawings of it in my diary look like a child's. As the sun rose behind the hospital, I kept my eyes on the moon, trying to fix it in my vision until it disappeared. It wavered, vanished, and reappeared three times before it was gone for good.

As the day broke, my view was of an enormous complex of hospital buildings, each painted in what was meant to be a cheerful pastel. The bright walls came to an abrupt end at flat black asphalt roofs, which were covered with trash. I could tell that the wind was blowing, because plastic bags filled with air floated to and fro over the rooftops all day long. I focused on the plastic bags, wondering whence they had come, what they had held, and in what part of the Gulf of Mexico they would strangle which wildlife. Turning my eyes downward I noticed people, coming and going, also in bright colors. I must have been above a staff entrance, since almost everyone who entered or exited beneath me was wearing scrubs.

Only a few were physicians. Although I had entered the hospital as an emergency case and had been tested for lethal disorders, I didn't see very many doctors inside the building, either. During the first half day, in an emergency department hallway, I had seen one doctor for three minutes; she gave me a nice sense of the spectacular death that my symptoms might presage. I saw a second doctor during my spinal tap, if being on my stomach with a needle in my back counts as seeing. Radiologists did read my scans, though I saw neither them nor their reports. One hospitalist talked to me for five minutes and another for four, and I saw a neurologist for fifteen minutes over Skype (the nervous system cannot be examined over Skype). This isn't much, but it is typical. In American hospitals, no one doctor ever seems to be responsible for a case, and patients strain to talk to anyone with authority.

We have an imbalance between the technique of tests and the technique of conversation. Of course, it is possible to err too far in the other direction, as Germans and Austrians sometimes do, and righteously avoid tests and medication (especially antibiotics) that really are necessary. My son had bacterial pneumonia in Vienna last spring, and it was a real struggle to persuade the doctors to test him for a bacterial infection. Like me, he did not complain enough, and male doctors did not take his mother seriously enough, so a system based on talking failed. That said, once the diagnosis was made, he was kept in the hospital as long as necessary, with attentive and superior care from doctors and nurses, and with no charges to us. He was admitted on his ninth birthday to the hospital where he was born, and the nurses and doctors made a fuss about that.

When I got sick in Munich last December, I also needed to complain more, and the doctors should have relied more on technology. If the German doctors had ordered a CT scan they would likely have seen a swollen appendix, and proceeded from there with antibiotics or surgery. That said, if I had been treated in Germany, I would have stayed much longer in hospital, been given appropriate antibiotics, and been observed. The cut-rate American disaster of being expelled right after an appendectomy without information about a second infection would have been impossible and indeed unthinkable. It was that scenario which brought me, ignorant of my own condition, to the hospital in Florida.

Although physicians were in short supply, what the Florida hospital did have in impressive numbers were elderly volunteers in khaki shorts and baseball caps. They were always ready, with a friendly wave, to drive patients from one pastel structure to another on speedy white golf carts. They also visited the patients in their rooms and asked how they could be helpful. It turns out that my default mode during medical treatment is polite and accommodating; when a volunteer asked about my experience at the hospital, I said that everything was just fine. The one thing I might mention, I said, was that I had hardly seen any physicians. I added that the nurses and the nurse assistants never seemed to know when doctors would make their rounds, or even who was on duty.

"You'd be surprised," the nice old gentleman said, "but that's what everyone says."

❧❧

The problem is not that doctors do not want to work with patients. As we see during the coronavirus pandemic, physicians can work extraordinarily hard and risk their own lives trying to save the lives of others. The problem is that doctors have very little say in what happens around them, and waste their time and energy pacifying greater powers. They no longer have the authority that patients expect and need. Every day, physicians have to pretend to patients that they matter more than they do. If patients understood how enserfed doctors have become, they would be less likely to come to hospitals, and less money would be made. American doctors are becoming props in advertisements, the front men and women whose coached smiles are meant to cover the gaps in our ragged patchwork of competing hospitals.

The pandemic was a moment when the cover dropped, when we could see that doctors do not matter in society and politics. The coronavirus was a financial bonanza for people with unrelated economic interests, such as owners of commercial real estate. The floodgates were opened for firms working for the Trump presidential campaign and companies whose owners donated to it. The richest zip code in America was granted two million dollars for no very clear reason. Insurance companies and private equity firms had a voice in policy; physicians and patients had none.

Though the economic crash of 2020 was actually a public health crisis, no doctors were convened to make recommendations. When the bailout was negotiated, we saw very few doctors and nurses on television proposing how the money might be spent. Our federal government managed to spend two trillion dollars without purchasing what we actually needed: tests, masks, gowns, and ventilators. Into early March it was actually the policy of the Trump administration to export masks made in this country to China. Not a single shipment of medical-grade N95 masks arrived on American shores in March 2020.

I am still in treatment and undergoing tests, so I see some of the consequences of this. It made me nervous to undergo an ultrasound carried out by a coughing, maskless technician. If doctors had been in charge, there would not have been such scenes. There would have been no plague in the first place, since we would have made testing a priority from the beginning. If doctors had authority, they would not have been trying to fight a pandemic without the necessary equipment. If doctors had sway, they would not have been wading into rooms full of infectious disease, day after day for months, without an appropriate number of masks.

A neighbor across the street, a physician with three

small children who was treating covid patients at the local hospital, used our block email list to ask if anyone could spare masks: "the hospital is out of small N95 masks (my size)." Even in the better-equipped hospitals, of which hers was one, doctors were getting a mask per week, when a mask is supposed to be disposable. They put their masks in brown paper bags with their names on them when they went home, and picked them up again the next day. Doctors in South Korea looked like they were coming from a science fiction movie; ours looked like they were coming from the Salvation Army.

Throughout the country, people working in hospitals were exposed to the virus far more than they should have been. Without testing and proper personal protective equipment they faced risks they could neither estimate nor avoid. They could not speak openly about these dangers, because the owners of private hospitals protected their brand. In commercial medicine, doctors are supposed to be flat smiling pixelated faces on billboards and in-house promotion videos, not real people with real concerns about patients' bodies—and their own. Doctors and nurses were fired for bringing their own protective gear to work, since this revealed that hospitals' stocks were inadequate. Commercial medicine halted free speech. We heard much less than we should have about these outrages because doctors and nurses were under gag orders from their employers. The president of the American Medical Association had to plea for "physicians' freedom to advocate for the best interest of their patients."

When I was very sick I spoke often with my father-in-law, a physician. In addition to his private practice, hospital rounds, and teaching rounds, he is also the responsible physician at a nursing home in Pennsylvania. He caught the disease there; a caregiver in the same facility died of it, as did eleven patients. His wife had a debilitating stroke—a result, it seems, of a blood clot related to covid-19. She could not get a test, so it is impossible to know for sure. What I can say for sure is that she no longer remembers the names of her grandchildren.

When Ohio started testing, a fifth of the positive results were from medical personnel. Doctors died all over the country: among them a beloved physician in a public hospital who chose to take risks to treat covid patients, and an emergency room physician who killed herself after seeing too many deaths by coronavirus.

Nurses died as well: a nurse who worked in a prison; a nurse who was tending to a colleague ill with the virus; a nurse whose daughter thought he was invincible; a nurse whose daughter texted desperately that "none of us can live without you." The first known victim in St. Louis was an African American nurse. Nurse assistants, technicians, paramedics, patient transporters: all of them got sick. When I was in the hospital I thought that the cleaning staff were probably doing the single most important job. They got sick, too. A janitor who was a Gulf War veteran died.

Older veterans died by the dozen in nursing homes. Mr. Trump kept calling the plague a "war," which raised the question of how many viruses our $700 billion in annual military spending stopped (zero). Money for the common defense would be better spent on public health. Mr. Trump's comparison to war was flawed, since it made his authoritarian incompetence seem like the result of some unexpected enemy attack. But if this is a war, it is one where the commander in chief ignored every warning and then sent troops to the front line without weapons and body armor. It is a war whose soldiers have no right to speak about what they saw; a war not of a silent generation, but of a silenced generation. It is a war that took more American lives than any since the Second World War—and even that could change.

⁂

When I got sick, it was hard to stay in the hospital long enough for proper diagnosis and treatment. My first three hospital stays each lasted a single night. If any of them had lasted just a day longer, my condition would likely have been diagnosed and treated sooner, and I would never have come so close to death. Every time I was in an American hospital, I felt the pressure to leave. In the lobby of the hospital on the night I nearly died there was no sense of concern, let alone welcome. Even in the emergency room on December 29th, I felt a weird atmosphere building. The next day, when I could move a bit, I wrote in my diary: "They said exhaustion. Flu? Give you some fluids. Wanted me out? Today they say sepsis."

Commercial medicine means tension over bed space. When the coronavirus plague reached the United States, we did not have enough hospital beds. This might seem strange at first: aren't epidemics regular events, and might there not be many occasions when more beds are needed than are regularly used? The reason why there are never excess beds, the reason why Americans who have appendectomies go home too soon, the reason why mothers are expelled prematurely from maternity wards, is that we have commercial medicine. The fundamental calculation is financial.

To understand the shortage of beds, it helps to think of just-in-time delivery. Companies like to have just enough space for what they need, work with, and sell, not more and not less. For a hospital, the human body is the object that is to be delivered, altered, and shipped away just in time. There should never be too many bodies, or too few bodies. There should be just the right number of bodies on just the right number of beds. Good doctors, good nurses, and good assistants resist this logic all the time, but they are pushing a boulder up a mountain.

Maintaining beds costs money. No hospital, in American commercial medicine, is going to maintain a reserve of beds when other hospitals do not do so. Since financial logic dominates medical logic, the country must always be unprepared for epidemics. There can never be a reserve of beds, nor for that matter a reserve of protective equipment or ventilators.

Managers counting on a quarterly profit cannot factor in pandemics, which arrive about once a decade. Each time a plague comes, the situation will be defined as exceptional, and the shortages will make the emergency even worse than it had to be. Then money will fly around: not to where the doctors might want, since they will not be asked, but to the sectors of the economy with the loudest voices. This just happened, and with commercial medicine it will keep happening.

In the hospital, sad to say, a body is a widget. Kindly assistants, competent nurses, and decent physicians try to humanize the widget, but they are constrained by a system. A body creates revenue if the body is the right kind of sick for the right length of time. Certain kinds of illnesses, especially ones treatable (or reputed to be treatable) with surgery and drugs, make money. No one has an economic incentive to keep you healthy, to get you well, or for that matter to keep you alive. Health and life are human values, not financial ones; an unregulated market in the treatment of our bodies generates profitable sickness rather than human thriving.

To be sure, many people in hospitals do care about health; I know that from the doctors who told me the truth, the nurses who stopped to give me advice and encouragement, the technicians who explained what tests meant, the transporters who gamely kept up the small talk while pushing my bed, the assistant who found a way to tie my liver bag so that I could walk, the cleaners who adjusted their schedules so that my floor wouldn't be slippery when I was trying to get out of bed. But hospitals as institutions have an incentive to get you out the door when the revenue stream declines, which is not the same thing as an incentive to return you to health. Insurance companies have an incentive not to pay for your tests and treatment.

Every time you are seen by a doctor or a nurse, every time a test is run, the algorithms of the hospital duel with the algorithms of the insurance company to see who will make how much money. Hospitals will tend to carry out procedures that are profitable, regardless of whether they have the best personnel on hand. If, for example, your newborn has a complicated heart defect, the local children's hospital might not direct you to the surgeon in another hospital who can best perform the demanding procedure, but will likely claim that its own surgeons are up to the task—even when this is not true. Babies then suffer and die.

At the other end of life, surgical implants provide a further example of where commercial medicine can place profit over health. I first became aware of them when my doctoral supervisor had his hip replaced. This senior historian had seen a great deal in life: he was a Holocaust survivor, the son of Wanda; it was on his desk that I saw her portrait for a quarter of a century. He lived in communist Poland, where he had helped to organize an underground university; he was interned in a camp under martial law.

For most of the time I knew him he was very fit, and skied each winter. When I visited him in the hospital after his surgery I thought that his hip replacement augured better mobility. In fact, he suffered more afterwards than before, never walked properly again, and died exhausted by pain.

In the United States, implants are essentially unregulated. We do not keep a register of which objects are in which bodies. Because legal standards are as lax as regulatory ones, we do not even learn from lawsuits about suffering and death caused by implants going wrong. It is likely that implants are one of the leading causes of death in the United States, perhaps even the single leading cause. But they make money.

Another conflict between the profit motive and the healing mission arises in the treatment of infections. The sepsis that nearly killed me was a bacterial infection. Once the bacterium was identified, I could be treated with the appropriate antibiotic, which cleared my blood of infection. My liver abscess is a bacterial infection, so I take an antibiotic. Unfortunately, bacteria evolve to gain resistance to antibiotics, which means that new antibiotics are constantly needed. Tens of thousands of Americans already die each year because antibiotic resistance has made their infections intractable. Yet since resistance means that new antibiotics might become obsolete, pharmaceutical companies hesitate to invest in developing them.

The worse the problem of antibiotic resistance becomes, the less hard the market works to find the solutions. Most of the big pharmaceutical companies no longer research antibiotics at all. If pure capitalist logic is applied to health, the bacteria win.

❧ ❧

The specialists in profit have made their way into the physical and mental space that was once controlled by the specialists in medicine. As computer programs determine how many patients can be profitably squeezed into a day, doctors become tools. Then the actual machines march triumphantly into the wards. Nurses are now separated from patients by computers on wheels that roll everywhere with them: their bossy robot taskmasters. When you first see a nurse, she or he will likely have eyes on the screen rather than on you. This has dreadful consequences for your treatment, since you become a checklist rather than a person. If you are having a problem unrelated to what is on the screen, some nurses will have a hard time gathering themselves and paying attention. For example, after my first liver procedure my liver drain was improperly attached. This was a serious problem that was easily reparable. Yet although I tried for four days to draw attention to it, I could not get through. It was not on the lists. And so I had a second liver procedure.

When I read my own medical record, I was struck by how often doctors wrote what was convenient rather than what was true. It's hard to blame them: they are locked in a terrible record-keeping system that sucks away their time and our money. When doctors enter their records, their hands are guided by the possible entries in the digital system, which are arranged to maximize revenue. The electronic medical record offers none of the research benefits that we might expect from its name; it is electronic in the same sense that a credit card reader or an ATM is electronic. It is of little help in assembling data that might be useful for doctors and patients. During the coronavirus pandemic, doctors could not use it to communicate about symptoms and treatments. As one doctor explained, "Notes are used to bill, determine level of service, and document it rather than their intended purpose, which was to convey our observations, assessment, and plan. Our important work has been co-opted by billing."

Doctors hate all of this. Doctors of an older generation say that things were better in their time—and, what is more worthy of note, younger doctors agree with them. Doctors feel crushed by their many masters and miss the authority that they used to enjoy, or that they anticipated that they would enjoy when they decided to go to medical school. Young people go to medical school for good reasons, then find their sense of mission exploited by their bosses. Pressured to see as many patients as possible, they come to feel like cogs in a machine. Hassled constantly by companies that seek to pry open every aspect of medical practice for profit, they find it hard to remember the nobility of their calling. Tormented by electronic records that take as much time as patient care, and tortured by mandatory cell phones that draw them away from thinking, they lose their ability to concentrate and communicate. When doctors are disempowered, we do not learn what we need to be healthy and free.

❦ ❦

During the pandemic it was difficult to get medical care of any kind, because the hospitals were reorganized to treat the novel coronavirus. The lack of equipment killed those infected by the coronavirus and those who treated them. Our shortages also killed countless people who did not have their cancer surgeries or organ transplants—or who just needed to see a doctor at the beginning of some malady that should never have developed further but, in the absence of care, did. Because hospitals could not perform profitable operations during the pandemic, they fired doctors just when patients needed them the most.

Why are big hospitals so central to basic care? In commercial medicine, hospitals are designed for "providers" (doctors, nurse practitioners, physician assistants) to supply certain deliverables at a certain price. But health is mainly a matter of education and prevention, tasks more easily accomplished away from hospitals. Wouldn't we all be healthier if we had a broader spectrum of public health and access to physicians throughout the country, and even at home? Physician visits to households prevent illness and encourage people to continue their treatments. People feel better when they can see a doctor personally. Doctors should work from thousands of small offices around the country, or even make house calls. Why does easy contact with a physician seem like a dream?

The pressure and complication of insurance and record keeping force doctors to form groups. These groups are then purchased by private equity firms to form larger staffing companies, or purchased by hospitals, which are then purchased by other hospitals. Regional oligopolies swallow whatever is in reach, as private equity firms race to make a profit before moving on. Whether a hospital was adequately staffed during the coronavirus pandemic had to do with national balance sheets, not local needs. None of this has anything to do with the basic labor of being a doctor. As

Benjamin Franklin wrote in another context, "the Malady consists in the *enormous Salaries, Emoluments, & Patronage* of great Offices."

A doctor who wants to work on her own within the community has to have a sense of mission, has to be prepared to earn less money—and has to have help. The life goal of a family friend in Ohio was to be a community doctor. And she managed to do this for a time, but only because her highly educated, math-oriented, and computer-literate husband made it his full-time job to deal with insurance and records. That is obviously not practicable for everyone.

※ ※

People need doctors close to home. People need doctors whom they know, who know them, who can follow their story, who can take charge in a crisis, who will feel responsible. We need a health care system that begins where people live, rather than expecting them to know everything themselves, or to master complicated paperwork, or to pay hidden fees.

Access to medical care is a problem in cities, where the emergency room becomes the first and only resort. Yet care is even more difficult to find across great swaths of the countryside and exurbia, where physicians are scarce and hospitals are distant. About 120 hospitals have closed in rural America in the past decade. Two of them shut their doors in March 2020, during the pandemic. Americans in rural counties without hospitals were more likely to die once infected. The first person known to have died of a novel coronavirus infection in West Virginia had just lost her local hospital.

As hard as it is to make it as a community doctor in the cities and the suburbs, it is all but impossible beyond them. It is not that doctors do not want that kind of work; some of them dream of it. It is just difficult to make a living advising and healing people one at a time. Specialists make more money than generalists, and young American doctors usually have debt. As a result, too few decide to become pediatricians and internists. The entire field of geriatrics, care for the old, is disappearing.

One of the reasons specialists make more money than general practitioners is that surgery is easier to bill, and easier to charge to insurance companies, than primary care. Yet primary care is what matters most for our health and especially for the health of our children. Once again, what is profitable is not what is healthy.

The novel coronavirus has made all of this worse. People are choosing not to see their primary care physicians, with the consequence that many small practices will close. The government bailout focused on entities irrelevant to medicine; the medical institutions that got attention were big hospitals. This means that the doctors who matter most are at risk of being driven out. The coronavirus could lead to even more centralized commercial medicine, which is the opposite of what Americans need.

If we value health, we can change what is profitable. It should not be hard to heal people one at a time. Doctors are not perfect, as I have had occasion to note. But in a better system a poor doctor becomes a mediocre one, a mediocre doctor becomes decent, a decent one becomes good, and a good one becomes outstanding. Doctors are the people who are trained in both the science and the humanism of care. When we think of medicine, we think of them, rather than of the corporations that hide behind their images on billboards. If we gave doctors the authority they deserve, we would all be healthier and freer.

Huge medical groups should be broken up by antitrust legislation. Doctors who provide primary care in underserved areas should have their debts forgiven. Gag orders of physicians should be made illegal. Doctors should be put in charge of revived federal agencies tasked with planning for and responding to epidemics. And doctors should be convened to help design a system in which all Americans are insured and have access to the care we need.

CONCLUSION

Our Recovery

We see our malady all too vaguely. We lack the local news that would help us focus on the countryside, on neighborhoods, on reality. The hospital billboards along our highways and the pharmaceutical ads on our television screens give us an upbeat message about technology despite our worsening malady. It matters that we have a procedure or a drug. Yet it matters more to have knowledge about our problems, doctors entrusted with authority, time to spend with our children, and a right to health care. No amount of propaganda can blur the basic fact about American commercial medicine: we pay a huge premium for the privilege of dying younger.

The medical industrial complex will defend our malady as the only possible reality. The lobbyists, the PR specialists, and their unholy host of internet memes will tell us that we cannot afford change. It is just too expensive, they will say, to listen to doctors, to rear children humanely, to find truth, to enjoy health. We will be instructed that freedom means its opposite: subjecting our bodies to the principle that someone somewhere who knows nothing about medicine and cares nothing about us should make as much money from our bodies with as little effort as possible. A free country, we are to understand, is one where ever fewer people extract ever more wealth from ever sicker American bodies.

This is a lie.

The idea that commercial medicine is efficient, even in simple economic terms, is grotesque. It is ludicrous to claim that our present system is cost effective. We pay far more for health care than do people in comparable countries, and we get far less. A failure in public health, the coronavirus epidemic, cost taxpayers trillions of dollars and crushed the entire economy. Let us remember that. Allowing people to fall ill is profitable for certain sectors—the ones who will defend the present system—but it makes the country poorer and the economy smaller. The declining health of millennials means sadder decades ahead for them, shorter and poorer retirements for Generation X, and less prosperity for everyone.

Health care that is too expensive is health care that does not work. Nearly half of Americans avoid medical treatment because they cannot pay for it. Tens of millions of Americans remain uninsured, and tens of millions more have insurance that is inadequate. I had decent health insurance, but still had to pay thousands of dollars in unexpected fees. Because I was still in the hospital when the bills began to arrive, I was charged penalties on fees that should not have existed in the first place. This financial chicanery makes us all sick.

Of course, it is much worse than this. During the coronavirus epidemic, tens of millions of Americans lost their insurance because they lost their jobs. All Americans then suffered because the unemployed were left behind. Since they were undiagnosed they spread the disease, and since they were untreated they suffered and died. Because we offer appallingly little sick leave everyone in the country was put at risk. People went to work while ill so as not to lose their jobs, and spread the infection. All of this is distinctly abnormal and entirely avoidable.

Solitude and solidarity need to be rebalanced. One reason that we are too lonely in this country is that we do not know how to talk about what ails us. If being a patient did not occasion anxieties about money and status, we would be more likely to get treated and get well. If we all had access to doctors and nurses whom we trusted, we would find it easier not just to get by but also to get along.

A right to health care is a foundation for better treatment and longer life, but also a step forward to a more just society in which we are all more free. If being a doctor were a calling rather than a subordinate position, if the rules were changed so that small practices could compete with the giants, we would all be healthier. We would move away from a politics of pain. The anxiety and the fear are not necessary. Our malady is curable.

Solidarity means that everyone takes part, rather than some people opting out. A source of our malady is the drastic inequality of wealth that separates the experiences of a very small group from everyone else. As Plato knew, this is how democracy becomes oligarchy, rule by the rich. When money becomes the only goal, values disappear, and people imitate the oligarchs. We do this now when we admire oligarchs' fantasies of immortality rather than ask why our own lives must be shortened. When we indulge the daydreams of the ultra-wealthy, we create what Plato called "a city of the rich" and "a city of the poor." When we turn a public health crisis into a bonanza for billionaires, we deepen our malady. When we overlook the offshored billions of our oligarchs, we miss our chance to make Americans healthier and freer. Even as more than twenty million Americans lost their jobs in the first weeks of the coronavirus pandemic, America's billionaires increased their combined wealth by two hundred and eighty-two billion dollars.

We should regard health care as a right, take medical and local knowledge seriously, make time for young children, and put doctors in charge. The realization of these lessons will cost some money now—and save far, far more in the years to come. The question is not how much this would cost. The question is how enormous the gains would be. Robust public health lowers medical costs and reduces the risk of pandemics that destroy the economy. Investing in childhood means less mental and physical illness down the road, less prison time, fewer broken lives. It means more wealth for those who retire.

Most of the insurance industry simply collects rents from disease, like trolls on a bridge demanding a toll. The trolls' profits misleadingly count in gross national product, though they are supplying no good and performing no service. Economic logic says that the middleman should be removed when possible, and we know how it is possible in this case: with a single-payer system at the center of things, and private insurance at the margins. Countries where people live longer have shown that this works. Thousands of doctors have made the case for it. If we all cross the bridge to health together, the trolls cannot stop us.

A market economy such as ours works better when people are cared for. If it is liberty that we want, then we do not sacrifice human freedom to market dogma, but rather make markets work for freedom. The most influential of the market economists, Friedrich Hayek, opposed oligopoly, or ownership by a few, which he compared to Soviet central planning. Our medical-industrial complex is a set of oligopolies. Our big data industry is also a set of oligopolies. Hayek is right: they should be broken up. In his most famous work, *The Road to Serfdom*, Hayek worried about a "dispossessed middle class," which commercial medicine is now creating. He took for granted that in civilized countries everyone would have access to care: "The case for the state's helping to organize a comprehensive system of social insurance," as he wrote, "is very strong." He knew that "there is no contradiction between the state's providing greater security in this way and the preservation of individual freedom."

In fact, the right policies make us more free by making us more secure. This is especially true for children. Our country will be more free in the future if we create structures that allow us to spend time with our children now. In the meantime, the services and rights that we need to parent well would not distort the market but perfect it. It makes no sense for mothers and fathers of young children to quit their jobs and find new ones because they have inadequate parental leave, sick leave, and vacation time. This creates stress in their own lives, and also generates costs for employers. Skills are constantly and needlessly lost, and new costs accrue in the constant retraining. Employees who have the right to sick leave, parental leave, and vacation are happier and more productive. They are also more free.

What we take for granted can change quickly and for the better. It can also change quickly and for the worse. Now we choose. It is easy to give money to the wrong people during a pandemic, and easy to give away freedom at any time. It takes work to be free, and courage to see opportunity. This crisis is a chance to rethink the possible. Health care should be a right, doctors should have authority, truth should be pursued, children should see a better America.

Let us begin our recovery.

Rage and Empathy

Even when the worst of the infection was behind me, it was weeks before I could sleep at night. My hands and feet still tingled, and my right side hurt from the operations. I was awakened by nurses and by worries. During long January nights in the hospital, I thought of home: the New England city where I live, and the part of the Midwest I come from. So that I could listen to music, my wife bought earphones and dug out an old black cell phone, its glass shattered years ago on a cobblestone in Kyiv. Now, when I feel better, I listen to music I hadn't known before; but in the hospital room, behind the closed shade, amidst the machines, with tubes in my arm and chest, I wanted to hear something familiar.

So I spent nights with Lucinda Williams, listening to *Car Wheels on a Gravel Road*. The title track recalled to me the breadth of our country, from my urban hospital bed near the Atlantic Ocean and Interstate 95 to all the little places westward and southward where the asphalt ends. I thought of the sound of the tires of a pickup on gravel, which I heard very distinctly as a child riding in an open bed, looking for deer in cornfields. The song is about going away in a hurry and in sadness; a child has dirt mixed with tears on her face. It is a song about pain. I drive a red pickup, a 1992 Dodge, which belonged to my father's father. It keeps me company on the East Coast. For me gravel roads are about coming back, the rattle and rumble of rubber on rock announcing a return, a recovery.

I am at home in New Haven now. I can't take my little girl to Ohio this spring as I promised her, because of the coronavirus pandemic, but at least I am alive and can think about a future that holds such prospects. This book began from some notes I made in my diary when I was raging against a final loneliness. I got the few more weeks that I craved then, and so I wrote. I still have a hole in my liver, though it is smaller now. Livers heal. Most likely mine is no longer infected; I will find out when I go off the antibiotics. The nine holes in me are now a constellation of scars. The soles of my feet still tingle, as does my left hand, and especially my left forefinger. In a moment I will type the final period of this book with it: not as a sign of resignation, but as a mark of improvement.

Even after we recover, scars and symptoms remain as a legacy of malady. Recovery is not going back to the way things were. I am not exactly as I was. My English vocabulary came back in bursts, like rain from some friendly cloud; I speak and write a little differently now. My other languages were not affected; I spoke Polish while septic and half-conscious on the way from the airport to the hospital; when I look at my wife's texts, I see that after surgery I asked for carrots, celery, and French mystery novels. A fair portion of my body was shaved for surgeries, injections, tubes, and an electrocardiogram. Some of the hair that was black grew back white; some of the hair that was white grew back black. I used to go to sleep at night thinking about the first cup of coffee the next morning; now I don't even like the smell. The other day, as I was preparing to brief the United Nations Security Council in what was to be my first lecture in half a year, I realized that I no longer knew how to tie a tie.

History is never entirely behind us. We can learn from the aspirations and failures of previous selves and previous eras, and create something new. I will not again be as I was before, nor do I wish to be; I have learned, and so I am better. I am still angry: not so much for myself as for all of us. We deserve freedom, and we need medicine that works. It would begin from people wherever they are, in cities or far from them, near highways or on gravel roads. It would begin from the premise that we have a right to health care. Does that sound like a dream? Let it be the American one.

Wherever we live in this country, however we might fall ill, we are not things but people, and we thrive when we are treated as such. Each of us has a torch that rages against death. And each of us is a plank of a raft that floats through life with others. Health is our common vulnerability, and our shared chance to grow freer together. Healing our malady would enrich life, extend liberty, and allow us to pursue happiness, alone and together, in solitude and in solidarity. To be free we need our health, and for our health we need one another.

ACKNOWLEDGMENTS

In this book I describe an escape from a flawed medical system in which many others remain, in pernicious conditions made all the worse by a pandemic. I am grateful to the doctors, physician assistants, nurses, nurse assistants, technicians, transporters, cleaners, cafeteria workers, and fellow patients who shared a moment, a smile, or a thought. Julie Clark Ireland and her family looked after me in Florida. Izabela Kalinowska drove me to the hospital in Connecticut. Dr. Stephen Shore helped me understand my illness while facing challenges of his own. Tina Bennett reached out at a difficult time, and Sharon Volckhausen came to visit. Daniel Markovits, Sarah Bilston, Stefanie Markovits, and Ben Polak were loyal friends. Tamar Gendler and Daniel Fedorowycz looked after my work when I could not. I thank my students for writing under adversity and setting a good example. Sara Silverstein got me thinking about health and history. Leah Mirakhor and Dr. Navid Hafez asked me to write this book. Tracy Fisher helped me through the practicalities, and Will Wolfslau and Aubrey Martinson gracefully moved the manuscript towards publication. Tim Duggan has been the best of editors, sympathetic, wise, and trustworthy. Elizabeth Bradley, Amanda Cook, Laura Donna, Susan Ferber, Dr. Arthur Lavin, Julie Leighton, Christine Snyder, Dr. E. E. Snyder, Leora Tanenbaum, and Dmitri Tymoczko read drafts. Julianne Kaphar brought me soup, and Titus Kaphar understood what I meant. Jason Stanley ran with me when I couldn't run alone. Erin Clark, Milena Lazarkiewicz, Shakila McKnight, Gina Panza, Chelsea Roncato, and Sarah Walters taught my children. Kalev and Talia Snyder were not distractions from this book but its source. Emile and Alain Stanley were their good friends. I thank Dr. Njeri Thande for being there, and Marci Shore for getting me home.

NOTES

PROLOGUE: SOLITUDE AND SOLIDARITY

4   **letter from prominent Bostonians** "Comtee of Boston About Abuse of the Town in England 1770," available online in the National Archives.

4   **"our public malady"** Madison to Jefferson, April 4, 1800, available online in the National Archives.

5   **America could become a free country** The lecture was recorded: www.dialoguesondemocracy .com/copy-of-timothy-snyder; I begin at 11:00.

INTRODUCTION: OUR MALADY

13   **life expectancy of Americans has declined** Lenny Bernstein, "U.S. Life Expectancy Declines Again," *Washington Post*, November 29, 2018.

13   **Black women often die** Linda Villarosa, "Why America's Black Mothers and Babies Are in a Life-or-Death Crisis," *New York Times*, April 11, 2018.

14   **millennials will live shorter lives** "The Economic Consequences of Millennial Health," Moody's Analytics for Blue Cross Blue Shield, 2019.

14   **incidentally involves some health care** I borrow this phrase from Peter Bach: "The Policy, Politics, and Law of Cancer," conference at the Yale Law School, February 9, 2018.

18   **"The whole history"** Frederick Douglass, "West Indian Emancipation," speech, August 3, 1857.

1. HEALTH CARE IS A HUMAN RIGHT.

21   **perhaps because the friend** The American Medical Association collects information on racial and other disparities in health care on its website.

26   **I wanted to speak to him** See lesson nine of *On*

Tyranny: Twenty Lessons from the Twentieth Century (New York: Tim Duggan Books, 2017).

30 **misreported them** I know that results were misreported because I have read my medical record.

31 **poorer at almost every task** On cell phones and concentration, see Adrian F. Ward et al., "Brain Drain: The Mere Presence of One's Own Smartphone Reduces Available Cognitive Capacity," *Journal of the Association for Consumer Research 2*, no. 2 (2017); Seungyeon Lee et al., "The Effects of Cell Phone Use and Emotion-Regulation Style on College Students' Learning," *Applied Cognitive Psychology*, June 2017.

33 **Someone had finally looked** This is not just my supposition; I've read my medical record and the timing is clear.

35 **easier to see fellow citizens** These are themes that I discussed with Tony Judt in *Thinking the Twentieth Century* (New York: Penguin, 2012). I am making the case that what we take to be natural—competition for health care—is in fact artificial. For a broader argument along these lines, see Rutger Bregman, *Humankind* (New York: Little, Brown, 2020).

37 **deliberate deprivation of health** These include a group of east European physicians active in the cause of international public health after the First World War. I borrow the term *commercial medicine* from one of them, Andrija Štampar. See George Vincent Diary, July 18, 1926, Rockefeller Foundation Archives, RG 12. I owe the reference to Sara Silverstein, who is completing a book on these doctors.

38 **first antisemitic letter** On this letter and its context see Timothy Snyder, "How Hitler Pioneered Fake News," *New York Times*, October 16, 2019. My account of Hitler's worldview can be found in *Black Earth* (New York: Tim Duggan Books, 2015). My other relevant book is *Bloodlands* (New York: Basic Books, 2010).

38 **Confining Jews in ghettos** Like most themes in Holocaust studies, illness in the ghetto was discussed by Raul Hilberg, *The Destruction of the European Jews* (New Haven, Conn.: Yale University Press, 2003), 1: 271–74.

39 **Another shelf of books** The standard account of the German camps is Nikolaus Wachsmann, *KL: A*

History of the Nazi Concentration Camps (New York: Farrar, Straus and Giroux, 2015).

39   **logic of reverse health care** Golfo Alexopoulos, *Illness and Inhumanity in Stalin's Gulag* (New Haven, Conn.: Yale University Press, 2017).

47   **onto something** "Sleep, nutrition, relationships," as a nurse once defined the fundaments of health care to me.

49   **main source of health information** C. Lee Ventola, "Direct-to-Consumer Pharmaceutical Advertising: Therapeutic or Toxic?" *P&T* 36, no. 10 (2011): 669. See also Ola Morehead, "The 'Good Life' Constructed in Direct-to-Consumer Drug Advertising," unpublished manuscript, 2018.

50   **slope is steeper now** Raj Chetty et al., "The Fading American Dream: Trends in Absolute Income Mobility Since 1940," *Science*, April 28, 2017.

50   **go it alone, without unions** Bruce Western and Jake Rosenfeld, "Unions, Norms, and the Rise in U.S. Wage Inequality," *American Sociological Review* 76, no. 4 (2011): 513–37; Jason Stanley, *How Fascism Works* (New York: Random House, 2018), chapter ten.

50   **Small farming is becoming untenable** Alana Semuels, "'They're Trying to Wipe Us Off the Map.' Small American Farmers Are Nearing Extinction," *Time*, November 27, 2019.

51   **now kill themselves in higher numbers** Matt Perdue, "A Deeper Look at the CDC Findings on Farm Suicides," National Farmers Union, blog, November 27, 2018; Debbie Weingarten, "Why Are America's Farmers Killing Themselves?" *Guardian*, December 11, 2018.

52   **One year, the eighty thousand** On Portsmouth, see Sam Quinones, *Dreamland: The True Tale of America's Opiate Epidemic* (London: Bloomsbury, 2016).

52   **White women in the South** Andrew Gelman and Jonathan Auerbach, "Age-Aggregation Bias in Mortality Trends," *Proceedings of the National Academy of Sciences*, February 16, 2016.

52   **The life expectancy** Anne Case and Angus Deaton, "Rising Morbidity and Mortality in Midlife Among White Non-Hispanic Americans in the 21st Century," *Proceedings of the National Academy of Sciences*, December 8, 2015.

53   **The one piece of information** J. Wasfy et al.,

"County Community Health Associations of Net Voting Shift in the 2016 U.S. Presidential Election," *PLOS ONE* 12, no. 10 (2017); Shannon Monnat, "Deaths of Despair and Support for Trump in the 2016 Presidential Election," Research Brief, 2016; Kathleen Frydl, "The Oxy Electorate," *Medium*, November 16, 2016; Jeff Guo, "Death Predicts Whether People Vote for Donald Trump," *Washington Post*, March 3, 2016; Harrison Jacobs, "The Revenge of the 'Oxy Electorate' Helped Fuel Trump's Election Upset," *Business Insider*, November 23, 2016.

53   **Desperate voters** See the discussion of sadopopulism in chapter six of my *The Road to Unfreedom: Russia, Europe, America* (New York: Tim Duggan Books, 2018); also, on pollution and self-sacrifice, see Arlie Hochschild, *Strangers in Their Own Land* (New York: The New Press, 2016).

55   **sadism to manslaughter** Jonathan M. Metzl, *Dying of Whiteness* (New York: Basic Books, 2019). The foundational text is W.E.B. Du Bois, *Black Reconstruction* (New York: Harcourt, Brace, 1935).

58   **the sadness in their correspondence** See, for example, Washington to Madison, October 14, 1793;

and Washington to Jefferson, October 11, 1793, both available online at the National Archives.

58 **impossible to summon Congress** In 1793 in Philadelphia. See also Danielle Allen, *Our Declaration* (New York: Liveright, 2014).

2. RENEWAL BEGINS WITH CHILDREN.

72 **an unequal start of life** Corinne Purtill and Dan Kopf, "The Class Dynamics of Breastfeeding in the United States of America," *Quartz*, July 23, 2017.

77 **scientists have to teach** For accessible introductions to the science, see the research briefs collected by the Center on the Developing Child at Harvard University.

78 **capacities that people need** C. Bethell et al., "Positive Childhood Experiences and Adult Mental and Relational Health in a Statewide Sample," *JAMA Pediatrics*, November 2019.

78 **interact with other people** It is useful to know that the founders of Amazon and Google attended schools where screens are not allowed, and that Steve Jobs kept his children away from his company's gadgets. Nicholas Kardaras, *Glow Kids* (New

York: St. Martin's Griffin, 2016), 22–32. No one I know in Silicon Valley sends their children to a school where screens are allowed. Even babysitters there are required to sign agreements not to bring the addictive products into the home. Nellie Bowles, "Silicon Valley Nannies Are Phone Police for Kids," *New York Times*, October 26, 2018.

78 **regulate emotions** Barbara Fredrickson, "The Broaden-and-Build Theory of Positive Emotions," *Philosophical Transactions of the Royal Society of London, Biological Sciences*, September 29, 2004, 1367–77.

78 **Without those positive emotions** V. Felitti et al., "The Relationship of Childhood Abuse and Household Dysfunction to Many of the Leading Causes of Death in Adults," *American Journal of Preventive Medicine*, May 1998, 245–58.

79 **intense and thoughtful attention** For a series of papers on the practice of childhood development, see "Advancing Early Childhood Development: From Science to Scale," *Lancet*, October 4, 2016.

79 **time is very hard to come by** Heather Boushey, *Finding Time* (Cambridge, Mass.: Harvard University Press, 2016).

85 **had disbanded** Laurie Garrett, "Trump Has Sabotaged America's Coronavirus Response," *Foreign Policy*, January 31, 2020; Oliver Milman, "Trump Administration Cut Pandemic Early Warning Program in September," *Guardian*, April 3, 2020; Gavin Yamey and Gregg Gonsalves, "Donald Trump: A Political Determinant of Covid-19," *British Medical Journal*, April 24, 2020; David Quammen, "Why Weren't We Ready for the Coronavirus?" *New Yorker*, May 4, 2020.

86 **last officer** Jimmy Kolker, "The U.S. Government Was Not Adequately Prepared for Coronavirus at Home or Abroad," *American Diplomat*, May 2020.

86 **surgeon general** Jerome Adams, tweet, February 1, 2020.

86 **novel coronavirus spread silently** Erin Allday and Matt Kawahara, "First Known U.S. Coronavirus Death Occurred on Feb. 6 in Santa Clara County," *San Francisco Chronicle*, April 22, 2020; Benedict Carey and James Glanz, "Hidden Outbreaks Spread Through U.S. Cities Far Earlier Than Americans Knew, Estimates Say," *New York Times*, April 23,

2020; Maanvi Singh, "Tracing 'Patient Zero': Why America's First Coronavirus Death May Forever Go Unmarked," *Guardian*, May 26, 2020.

86   **ignoring the warnings** Frank Harrington, "The Spies Who Predicted COVID-19," *Project Syndicate*, April 16, 2020.

86   **On January 24th, he praised China** Donald Trump, tweet, January 24, 2020.

87   **On February 7th, he renewed his praise** Donald Trump, tweet, February 7, 2020.

87   **cruise ship** Motoko Rich and Edward Wong, "They Escaped an Infected Ship, but the Flight Home Was No Haven," *New York Times*, February 17, 2020.

87   **a "miracle"** Maegan Vazquez and Caroline Kelly, "Trump Says Coronavirus Will 'Disappear' Eventually," CNN, February 27, 2020.

87   **secretary of commerce** Juliet Eilperin et al., "U.S. Manufacturers Sent Millions of Dollars of Face Masks, Other Equipment to China Early This Year," *Washington Post*, April 18, 2020. See also Aaron Davis, "In the Early Days of the Pandemic, the U.S. Government Turned Down an Offer to Manufacture Millions of N95 Masks in America," *Washington Post*, May 10, 2020.

87   **tens of millions** Lauren Aratani, "US Job Losses Pass 40m as Coronavirus Crisis Sees Claims Rise 2.1m in a Week," *Guardian*, May 28, 2020.

88   **"under control"** Donald Trump, tweet, February 24, 2020.

88   **three hundred and fifty-two people** Eric Topol, "US Betrays Healthcare Workers in Coronavirus Disaster," Medscape, March 30, 2020; Timothy Egan, "The World Is Taking Pity on Us," *New York Times*, May 8, 2020.

88   **would now rank among** According to the Johns Hopkins University Coronavirus Research Center, coronavirus.jhu.edu/us-map, webpage accessed May 27, 2020.

90   **Not wanting to know about disease** Yuval Harari made a similar point in "The World After Coronavirus," *Financial Times*, March 20, 2020. Hobbes put it this way: "Want of science, that is, ignorance of causes, disposeth, or rather constraineth, a man to rely on the advice and authority of others." Thomas Hobbes, *Leviathan*, ed. J.C.A. Gaskin (Oxford: Oxford University Press, 2008 [1651]), 69.

91   **associated with higher death rates** Joseph Magagnoli et al., "Outcomes of Hydroxychloroquine

Usage in United States Veterans Hospitalized with Covid-19," medRxiv, April 16, 2020; Mayla Gabriela Silva Borba et al., "Effect of High vs. Low Doses of Chloroquine Diphosphate as Adjunctive Therapy for Patients Hospitalized with Severe Acute Respiratory Syndrome Coronavirus 2 (SARS-CoV-2) Infection," *JAMA Network Open*, April 24, 2020; Toluse Olorunnipa, Ariana Eunjung Cha, and Laurie McGinley, "Drug Promoted by Trump as 'Game-Changer' Increasingly Linked to Deaths," *Washington Post*, May 16, 2020.

91 **A federal official who quite properly questioned** Michael D. Shear and Maggie Haberman, "Health Dept. Official Says Doubts on Hydroxychloroquine Led to His Ouster," *New York Times*, April 22, 2020; Joan E. Greve, "Ousted U.S. Government Scientist Files Whistleblower Complaint over Covid-19 Concerns," *Guardian*, May 5, 2020.

91 **Another who reported shortages** Peter Baker, "Trump Moves to Replace Watchdog Who Identified Critical Medical Shortages," *New York Times*, May 1, 2020.

91 **Mr. Trump then wondered aloud** David Smith, "Coronavirus: Medical Experts Denounce Trump's

Latest 'Dangerous' Treatment Suggestion," *Guardian*, April 24, 2020.

91 **since Plato** Plato, *The Republic*, book 9. The investigative reporting of Edward Lucas confirms this: "Inside Trump's Coronavirus Meltdown," *Financial Times*, May 14, 2020. Zeynep Tufekci made the same point about China's early response: "How the Coronavirus Revealed Authoritarianism's Fatal Flaw," *Atlantic*, February 22, 2020.

92 **On March 6th** Gabriella Borter and Steve Gorman, "Coronavirus Found on Cruise Ship as More U.S. States Report Cases," Reuters, March 6, 2020.

92 **thousands of needless deaths** "Remarks by President Trump and Vice President Pence at a Meeting with Governor Reynolds of Iowa," WhiteHouse .gov, May 6, 2020.

92 **On June 15th** Kate Rogers and Jonathan Martin, "Pence Misleadingly Blames Coronavirus Spikes on Rise in Testing," *New York Times*, June 15, 2020; Michael D. Shear, Maggie Haberman, and Astead W. Herndon, "Trump Rally Fizzles as Attendance Falls Short of Campaign's Expectations," *New York Times*, June 20, 2020.

93 **American racists portrayed blacks** Khalil Gibran

Muhammad, *The Condemnation of Blackness* (Cambridge, Mass.: Harvard University Press, 2019), especially chapter two.

94 **Russia claimed** Timeline of Russian propaganda in "Disinformation That Can Kill: Coronavirus-Related Narratives of Kremlin Propaganda," Euromaidan Press, April 16, 2020; see also the continuing work of EU vs. Disinfo, euvsdisinfo.eu.

94 **China soon said the same** Rikard Jozwiak, "EU Monitors See Coordinated COVID-19 Disinformation Effort by Iran, Russia, China," *RFE/RL*, April 22, 2020; Julian E. Barnes, Matthew Rosenberg, and Edward Wong, "As Virus Spreads, China and Russia See Openings for Disinformation," *New York Times*, March 28, 2020.

94 **The Republican Party** Alex Isenstadt, "GOP Memo Urges Anti-China Assault over Coronavirus," Politico, April 24, 2020.

95 **does bear responsibility** "China Didn't Warn Public of Likely Pandemic for 6 Key Days," Associated Press, April 15, 2020.

95 **Some of the most valiant people** Vaccination for smallpox began in England in the early nineteenth century, thanks to Edward Jenner. Another preven-

tive therapy, variolation, in which material from smallpox sores was given to healthy people, was known earlier in China, India, and the Ottoman Empire. Smallpox has now been eradicated by vaccination.

96 **we are part of nature** I make a similar argument with respect to climate change in *Black Earth*.

96 **riding the roiling emotions** Tony Judt talked with me about the politics of fear in *Thinking the Twentieth Century*.

97 **African Americans kept dying** The first twelve people to die in St. Louis were black. A black nurse died after her own hospital turned her away four times. African Americans were 40 percent of the first victims in Detroit, 67 percent in Chicago, 70 percent in Louisiana. See Ishena Robinson, "Black Woman Dies from Coronavirus After Being Turned Away 4 Times from Hospital She Worked at for Decades," *The Root*, April 26, 2020; Fredrick Echols, "All 12 COVID-19 Deaths in the City of St. Louis Were Black," *St. Louis American*, April 8, 2020; Khushbu Shah, "How Racism and Poverty Made Detroit a New Coronavirus Hot Spot," Vox, April 10, 2020. See also Sabrina Strings, "It's Not

Obesity. It's Slavery," *New York Times*, May 25, 2020; Rashad Robinson, "The Racism That's Pervaded the U.S. Health System for Years Is Even Deadlier Now," *Guardian*, May 5, 2020.

97   **requested the authority** Betsy Woodruff Swan, "DOJ Seeks New Emergency Powers amid Coronavirus Pandemic," Politico, March 21, 2020.

97   **fired inspectors general** Julian Borger, "Watchdog Was Investigating Pompeo for Arms Deal and Staff Misuse Before Firing," *Guardian*, May 18, 2020; Veronica Stracqualursi, "Who Trump Has Removed from the Inspector General Role," CNN, May 16, 2020.

97   **the problem with unimpeded voting** Donald Trump, *Fox and Friends*, March 30, 2020. For a thorough history of foreign intervention in democratic elections, see David Shimer, *Rigged* (New York: Knopf, 2020).

98   **"liberate"** Tweets of April 17, 2020.

98   **respond better to pandemics** Amartya Sen made this point about famines. On disease, see Thomas Bollyky et al., "The Relationships Between Democratic Experience, Adult Health, and Cause-Specific Mortality in 170 Countries Between 1980 and

2016," *Lancet*, April 20, 2019; also "Diseases Like Covid-19 Are Deadlier in Non-Democracies," *Economist*, February 18, 2020.

98 **get more of a voice** Shefali Luthra, "Trump Wrongly Said Insurance Companies Will Waive Co-pays for Coronavirus Treatments," Politifact, March 12, 2020; Carol D. Leonnig, "Private Equity Angles for a Piece of Stimulus Windfall," *Washington Post*, April 6, 2020.

99 **authoritarian leaders** Réka Kinga Papp, "Orbán's Political Product," *Eurozine*, April 3, 2020; Andrew Kramer, "Russian Doctor Detained After Challenging Virus Figures," *New York Times*, April 3, 2020; Andrew Kramer, "'The Fields Heal Everyone': Post-Soviet Leaders' Coronavirus Denial," *New York Times*, April 2, 2020; "Philippines: President Duterte Gives 'Shoot to Kill' Order amid Pandemic Response," Amnesty International, April 2, 2020; "In Turkmenistan, Whatever You Do, Don't Mention the Coronavirus," *RFE/RL*, March 31, 2020.

99 **die uncounted** The Chinese numbers seem unbelievable. Russia seems to be suppressing the number of dead. "MID RF prizval FT i NYT," *RFE/RL*, May 14, 2020; Matthew Luxmoore, "Survey: 1 in 3

166

Russian Doctors Told to 'Adjust' COVID-19 Stats," *RFE/RL*, May 22, 2020; Anna Łabuszewska, "Defilada zwycięstwa nad koronawirusem i czeczeński pacjent," *Tygodnik Powszechny*, May 23, 2020. See also: Manas Kaiyrtayuly, "Kazakh COVID-19 Cemetery Has More Graves Than Reported Coronavirus Victims," *RFE/RL*, May 25, 2020.

99   **little counting of cases** " 'It's Horrific': Coronavirus Kills Nearly 70 at Massachusetts Veterans' Home," *Guardian*, April 28, 2020; Candice Choi and Jim Mustian, "Feds Under Pressure to Publicly Track Nursing Home Outbreaks," Associated Press, April 15, 2020.

99   **Florida has suppressed data** Kathleen McGrory and Rebecca Woolington, "Florida Medical Examiners Were Releasing Coronavirus Death Data. The State Made Them Stop," *Tampa Bay Times*, April 29, 2020.

100   **excess deaths** Maggie Koerth, "The Uncounted Dead," FiveThirtyEight, May 20, 2020.

101   **Values such as life** For important discussions, see Shoshana Zuboff, *The Age of Surveillance Capitalism* (London: Profile Books, 2019); Franklin Foer, *World Without Mind* (New York: Penguin, 2017);

also Naomi Klein, "How Big Tech Plans to Profit from the Pandemic," *Guardian*, May 10, 2020.

101 **brought us very little** Big data can of course be used for purposes other than profit, but its use in health requires deliberate efforts that are only just beginning. For a balanced review, see Adrian Cho, "Artificial Intelligence Systems Aim to Sniff Out Signs of COVID-19 Outbreaks," *Science*, May 12, 2020.

101 **obese Americans are most at risk** Shikha Garg et al., "Hospitalization Rates and Characteristics of Patients Hospitalized with Laboratory-Confirmed Coronavirus Disease 2019—COVID-NET, 14 States, March 1–30, 2020," *CDC Morbidity and Mortality Weekly Report*, April 17, 2020; Bertrand Cariou et al., "Phenotypic Characteristics and Prognosis of Inpatients with COVID-19 and Diabetes: The CORONADO Study," *Diabetologia*, May 7, 2020.

102 **not our common needs** Safiya Umoja Noble, *Algorithms of Oppression* (New York, NYU Press, 2018); Virginia Eubanks, *Automating Inequality* (New York: St. Martin's, 2017).

102 **the knowledge that we need** We could tell which

cities were infected by the (creepy) covert mass collection of body temperatures from smart thermometers, but that was after the fact. See Edward Lucas, *Cyberphobia* (New York: Bloomsbury, 2015); Roger McNamee, *Zucked* (London: Penguin, 2019); Nicholas Carr, *The Shallows* (New York: W. W. Norton, 2011).

102 **aim at addiction** I discuss digital politics in "What Turing Told Us About the Digital Threat to a Human Future," *New York Review Daily*, May 6, 2019; and in the expanded German text *Und wie elektrische Schafe träumen wir. Humanität, Sexualität, Digitalität* (Vienna: Passagen, 2020). See Brett Frischmann and Evan Selinger, *Re-engineering Humanity* (Cambridge: Cambridge University Press, 2018); Jaron Lanier, *Ten Arguments for Deleting Your Social Media Accounts Right Now* (New York: Henry Holt, 2018); Martin Burckhardt, *Philosophie der Maschine* (Berlin: Matthes and Seitz, 2018).

103 **human daring** See Michel Foucault, "Discourse and Truth: The Problematization of Parrhesia," lectures of 1983, available at foucault.info; see also Kieran Williams, *Václav Havel* (London: Reaktion Books, 2016); Marci Shore, "A Pre-History of Post-

Truth, East and West," *Eurozine*, September 1, 2017.

104 **take the advertising revenue** See the discussion in Lee McIntyre, *Post-Truth* (Cambridge, Mass.: MIT Press, 2018), 80–118.

105 **wild falsehoods** Sheera Frenkel, Ben Decker, and Davey Alba, "How the 'Plandemic' Movie and Its Falsehoods Spread Widely Online," *New York Times*, May 20, 2020; Jane Lytvynenko, "The 'Plandemic' Video Has Exploded Online," Buzzfeed, May 7, 2020.

105 **Most of our country** See the continuing work of Penelope Muse Abernathy, www.usnewsdeserts .com; also Margaret Sullivan, *Ghosting the News* (New York: Columbia Global Reports, 2020).

105 **In Kentucky** Charles Bethea, "Shrinking Newspapers and the Costs of Environmental Reporting in Coal Country," *New Yorker*, March 26, 2019.

106 **excuse to legalize pollution** Katelyn Burns, "The Trump Administration Wants to Use the Coronavirus Pandemic to Push for More Deregulation," Vox, April 21, 2020; Emily Holden, "Trump Dismantles Environmental Protections Under Cover of Coronavirus," *Guardian*, May 11, 2020; Emily

Holden, "U.S. Lets Corporations Delay Paying Environmental Fines amid Pandemic," *Guardian*, May 27, 2020. Pollution seems to be one reason African Americans are dying of covid-19 at such high rates. See Linda Villarosa, "'A Terrible Price': The Deadly Racial Disparities of Covid-19 in America," *New York Times*, April 29, 2020.

107 **By inviting a new epidemic** William C. Becker and David A. Fiellin, "When Epidemics Collide: Coronavirus Disease 2019 (COVID-19) and the Opioid Crisis," *Annals of Internal Medicine*, April 2, 2020.

107 **portraits of those who died** An example: "Remembering Vermonters Lost to the Coronavirus," VTDigger. When rural authorities understood that a pandemic was under way, the absence of newspapers made it hard to communicate health guidelines.

108 **death of truth** See Snyder, *Road to Unfreedom*, as well as Peter Pomerantsev, *Nothing Is True and Everything Is Possible* (New York: Public Affairs, 2015); and Anne Applebaum, *Twilight of Democracy* (London: Penguin, 2020). Three points of reference are George Orwell's "The Politics of the English Lan-

guage" (1946), Hannah Arendt's "Truth and Politics" (1967), and Václav Havel's "The Power of the Powerless" (1978).

4. DOCTORS SHOULD BE IN CHARGE.

115 **As we see during the coronavirus pandemic** See Rivka Galchen, "The Longest Shift," *New Yorker*, April 27, 2020.

116 **ragged patchwork** Lovisa Gustafsson, Shanoor Seervai, and David Blumenthal, "The Role of Private Equity in Driving Up Health Care Prices," *Harvard Business Review*, October 29, 2019.

116 **firms working for the Trump presidential campaign** Stephen Gandel and Graham Kates, "Phunware, a Data Firm for Trump Campaign, Got Millions in Coronavirus Small Business Help," CBS News, April 23, 2020.

116 **companies whose owners donated** Lee Fang, "Small Business Rescue Money Flowing to Major Trump Donors, Disclosures Show," *Intercept*, April 24, 2020.

116 **richest zip code** Aaron Leibowitz, "Approved for $2M Federal Loan, Fisher Island Now Asking Res-

idents Whether to Accept It," *Miami Herald*, April 23, 2020.

116 **private equity firms had a voice** Pema Levy, "How Health Care Investors Are Helping Run Jared Kushner's Shadow Coronavirus Task Force," *Mother Jones*, April 21, 2020.

117 **Not a single shipment** Susan Glasser, "How Did the U.S. End Up with Nurses Wearing Garbage Bags?" *New Yorker*, April 9, 2020.

117 **A neighbor across the street** Marci Shore, interviewed by Michaela Terenzani, "American Historian: Our Enormous Wealth Means Little Without a Public Health System," *Slovak Spectator*, April 8, 2020.

119 **doctors and nurses were under gag orders** Theresa Brown, "The Reason Hospitals Won't Let Doctors and Nurses Speak Out," *New York Times*, April 21, 2020; Nicholas Kristof, "'I Do Fear for My Staff,' a Doctor Said. He Lost His Job," *New York Times*, April 1, 2020.

119 **American Medical Association** Patrice A. Harris, "AMA Backs Physician Freedom to Advocate for Patient Interests," April 1, 2020.

119 **When Ohio started testing** Dan Horn and Terry

DeMio, "Health Care Workers in Ohio Are Testing Positive for COVID-19 at an Alarming Rate," *Cincinnati Enquirer*, April 13, 2020.

119 **a beloved physician in a public hospital** Michael Schwirtz, "A Brooklyn Hospital Mourns the Doctor Who Was 'Our Jay-Z,'" *New York Times*, May 18, 2020.

119 **emergency room physician who killed herself** Ali Watkins et al., "Top E.R. Doctor Who Treated Virus Patients Dies by Suicide," *New York Times*, April 27, 2020.

120 **Nurses died as well** For a minimum count of 9,282 medical workers killed in the first eight weeks, see CDC, "Characteristics of Health Care Personnel with COVID-19—United States, February 12—April 9," April 17, 2020. See MedPage Today for a running list of medical workers killed.

120 **"none of us can live without you"** Michael Rothfeld, Jesse Drucker, and William K. Rashbaum, "The Heartbreaking Last Texts of a Hospital Worker on the Front Lines," *New York Times*, April 15, 2020.

120 **first known victim** Rebecca Rivas, "Nurse Judy Wilson-Griffin," *St. Louis American*, March 20, 2020.

120 **Gulf War veteran** See the *Guardian*'s "Lost on the Frontline" for this and further profiles.

120 **Older veterans died** Tracy Tulley, "'The Whole Place Is Sick Now': 72 Deaths at a Home for U.S. Veterans," *New York Times*, May 10, 2020.

122 **Maintaining beds costs money** Something similar can be said about ventilators. One reason why they ran short is that they are produced only in an expensive and complicated form. When the federal government tried to contract a company to build cheaper and simpler ventilators, it was purchased by another firm that made the costlier variety. See Shamel Azmeh, "The Perverse Economics of Ventilators," Project Syndicate, April 16, 2020.

123 **once a decade** The conquest of nature risks not only zoonotic epidemics such as HIV, SARS, MERS, and the novel coronavirus. The de facto reduction of earth's mammals to a few breeds of a few species creates ideal conditions for epidemics among the animals that feed us. Right now about 66 percent of all mammal biomass is domesticated livestock, and another 30 percent is human, meaning that all wild mammals taken together account for only about four percent. The arrival of African

swine fever in the United States is a matter of time. See Olivia Rosane, "Humans and Big Ag Livestock Now Account for 96 Percent of Mammal Biomass," EcoWatch, May 28, 2018; Greg Cima, "Guarding Against an Outbreak, Expecting Its Arrival," *JAVMA News*, May 1, 2020.

124 **complicated heart defect** Elizabeth Cohen, "10 Ways to Get Your Child the Best Heart Surgeon," CNN, August 4, 2013; Kristen Spyker, "Heterotaxy Syndrome," blog posts, March 11 and April 6, 2012.

125 **leading causes of death** Jerome Groopman, "The Cutting Edge," *New Yorker*, April 20, 2020; also his book *How Doctors Think* (New York: Houghton Mifflin, 2007), especially the sections on his own back surgery.

126 **no longer research antibiotics** Elizabeth Schumacher, "Big Pharma Nixes New Drugs Despite Impending 'Antibiotic Apocalypse,'" *Deutsche Welle*, September 14, 2019; "A Troubling Exit: Drug Company Ends Antibiotics Research," *Star-Tribune*, July 20, 2018.

128 **"Notes are used to bill"** Siddhartha Mukherjee, "What the Coronavirus Reveals About American Medicine," *New Yorker*, April 27, 2020.

130   **Physician visits to households** Katherine A. Orn-
      stein et al., "Epidemiology of the Homebound Pop-
      ulation in the United States," *JAMA Internal
      Medicine*, July 2015; Tina Rosenberg, "Reviving
      House Calls by Doctors," *New York Times*, Septem-
      ber 27, 2016.

130   **national balance sheets** Isaac Arnsdorf, "Over-
      whelmed Hospitals Face a New Crisis: Staffing
      Firms Are Cutting Their Doctors' Hours and Pay,"
      ProPublica, April 3, 2020.

131   **"the Malady consists"** Franklin to Henry Lau-
      rens, February 12, 1784, available online at the Na-
      tional Archives.

132   **About 120 hospitals have closed** Jack Healy et
      al., "Coronavirus Was Slow to Spread to Rural
      America. Not Anymore," *New York Times*, April 8,
      2020.

132   **Americans in rural counties** Suzanne Hirt, "Rural
      Communities Without a Hospital Struggle to
      Fight Rising Coronavirus Cases, Deaths," *USA
      Today*, May 15, 2020.

132   **The first person known** Healy et al., "Coronavirus
      Was Slow."

132   **too few decide** K. E. Hauer et al., "Factors Associ-

ated with Medical Students' Career Choices Regarding Internal Medicine," *Journal of the American Medical Association*, September 10, 2008, 1154–64.

132 **field of geriatrics** Atul Gawande, *Being Mortal* (New York: Macmillan, 2014), 36–48.

133 **doctors who matter most** Reed Abelson, "Doctors Without Patients: 'Our Waiting Rooms Are Like Ghost Towns,'" *New York Times*, May 5, 2020.

CONCLUSION: OUR RECOVERY

136 **we pay a huge premium** See Elizabeth H. Bradley and Lauren A. Taylor, *The American Health Care Paradox* (New York: Public Affairs, 2013).

137 **financial chicanery** These surprise charges are one way that private equity firms try to make a quick profit after buying hospitals and loading them down with debt; the result is that more people are shut out of health care.

137 **All Americans then suffered** Robert Reich, "Covid-19 Pandemic Shines a Light on a New Kind of Class Divide and Its Inequalities," *Guardian*, April 26, 2020.

139 **how democracy becomes oligarchy** Plato, *Repub-*

lic, book 8. See also Raymond Aron, *Dix-huit leçons sur la société industrielle* (Paris: Gallimard, 1962), 55.

139 **America's billionaires increased their combined wealth** Chuck Collins, Omar Ocampo, and Sophia Paslaski, "Billionaire Bonanza," Institute for Policy Studies, April 2020. See also Chris Roberts, "San Francisco Has 75 Billionaires. Most of Them Aren't Donating to Local COVID-19 Relief," *Curbed*, April 30, 2020.

140 **Thousands of doctors** See the resources on the website of Physicians for a National Health Care Program (PNHP), pnhp.org.

140 **most influential of the market economists** Friedrich Hayek, *The Road to Serfdom*, ed. Bruce Caldwell (Chicago: University of Chicago Press, 2017 [1944]), 207, 215, 148–49.

EPILOGUE: RAGE AND EMPATHY

146 **first lecture in half a year** It was recorded: www .youtube.com/watch?v=Ohljz-a1fZE&t=1191s; I begin at 20:45.

ABOUT THE AUTHOR

TIMOTHY SNYDER is the Levin Professor of History at Yale University and a Permanent Fellow at the Institute for Human Sciences in Vienna. His fifteen books have appeared in more than forty languages. They have been honored with the Hannah Arendt Award for Political Thought, the Leipzig Book Prize for European Understanding, the Literature Award of the American Academy of Arts and Letters, the award of the Dutch Auschwitz Committee, and the Warsaw Ghetto Uprising Medal, among other distinctions. His work has inspired paintings, posters, sculpture, plays, films, punk rock, rap, and opera. His words are quoted around the world in demonstrations in defense of freedom. He lives in New Haven, Connecticut.